Osteoporosis— The Silent Thief

William A. Peck, M.D., and
Louis V. Avioli, M.D.

An AARP Book
published by
American Association of Retired Persons, Washington, D.C.
Scott, Foresman and Company, Glenview, Illinois

AARP Books provides interesting, timely, and practical information that enables persons 50 and over to improve the quality of their lives in their health, housing, finances, recreation, personal relationships, and work environment. These books are copublished by AARP, the world's largest membership and service organization for people 50 and over, and Scott, Foresman and Company, one of the nation's foremost educational publishers. For further information, contact AARP Books, 1900 East Lake Avenue, Glenview, IL 60025.

Copyright © 1988
Scott, Foresman and Company, Glenview, Illinois
American Association of Retired Persons, Washington, D.C.
All Rights Reserved
Printed in the United States of America

Library of Congress Cataloging-in-Publication Data

Peck, William A. (William Arno), 1933–
  Osteoporosis.

  Bibliography: p.
  Includes index.
  1. Osteoporosis—Popular works. I. Avioli,
Louis V. II. Title.
RC931.073P43   1988   616.7'1   87-33471
ISBN 0-673-24837-2

Illustration on page 10 from *A Woman's Guide to Good Health After 50* by Marie Feltin, M.D. Copyright © by Scott, Foresman and Company and American Association of Retired Persons, 1987.

This publication is protected by Copyright and permission should be obtained from the publisher prior to any prohibited reproduction, storage in a retrieval system, or transmission in any form or by any means, electronic, mechanical, photocopying, recording, or otherwise. For information regarding permission, write to Scott, Foresman and Company, 1900 East Lake Avenue, Glenview, Illinois 60025.

● Contents

Acknowledgments *v*
Preface *vii*
1. Understanding Osteoporosis—An Overview *1*
2. Form and Function of Bones *8*
3. Fracture—A Hazard of Osteoporosis *13*
4. Bone Changes with Age *20*
5. Risk Factors—and Protective Factors—for Osteoporosis *31*
6. Medical Causes of Osteoporosis *43*
7. Measuring Bone Mass *50*
8. Strengthening Bone Through Diet *59*
9. Calcium Supplements *82*
10. Physical Exercise and Bone Health *86*
11. Estrogen Therapy (ET) After Menopause *96*
12. Nonestrogen Prevention and Treatment—Established and Experimental *109*
13. Living with Osteoporosis—How to Prevent Fractures *115*
14. New Thrusts in Current Research *123*
Bibliography *127*
Index *129*
About the Authors *133*

● Acknowledgments

Patricia Peck, James Havranek, and Elaine Goldberg made many invaluable contributions to this book. Mrs. Peck created the first drafts of the Preface, chapter 1, and chapter 13 and aided in their finalization. Mr. Havranek, of the Department of Medicine, Jewish Hospital at Washington University, provided thorough overall editing and helped prepare the final manuscript. Mrs. Goldberg, at Scott, Foresman and Company, directed the final editing of the work. We thank Dr. Ronald Strickler for his careful review of chapter 11, on estrogen therapy, and the many other medical specialists who read portions of the initial manuscript and provided valuable comments.

● Preface

Fictional cultures of the future are often described as having conquered disease and prolonged life. To a limited extent, that fiction has become fact. Improved food processing, better sanitation, enhanced nutrition, and the availability of vaccines and antibiotics have virtually erased many diseases that were commonplace in our society some fifty years ago. As a result, life expectancy has increased dramatically—reaching the heretofore unimaginable seventy-nine years for women and seventy-four years for men. Twelve percent of the United States population is now sixty-five years old or older, and that figure is expected to reach 20 percent by the year 2030. In fact, people seventy-five years old and older represent the most rapidly growing group in our society. But we have been thwarted in our efforts to achieve the disease-free life of science fiction. A longer life increases the risk of so-called aging-associated disorders—arthritis; vascular diseases of the heart, brain, and limbs; certain types of cancer; and Alzheimer's disease. Some are preventable—just elimination of cigarette smoking would sharply decrease certain cancers and the likelihood of vascular disorders—but most are not.

By contrast, osteoporosis is a serious, potentially preventable health problem that accompanies advancing age.

Literally meaning "porous bones," osteoporosis is a condition in which bones have lost so much tissue that they are easily broken. It afflicts as many as 25 million Americans and causes over 1.3 million fractures, or breaks in a bone—particularly fractures of the spine, hip, and wrist. It is responsible for deformity, pain, loss of independence, and death. Its cost is enormous—an estimated 10 billion dollars annually.

Osteoporosis is known as the silent thief—the end result of painless, gradual losses of bone tissue accompanying aging. By the time a bone breaks, much of the damage has been done.

Although recognized for centuries, osteoporosis has only recently become identified as a significant threat to health. A 1984 conference sponsored by the federal government (National Institutes of Health) publicized the frequency and seriousness of the condition; emphasized how it can and should be prevented; pointed out the roles of estrogen therapy, calcium, exercise, general nutrition, and other strategies in reducing bone loss; and suggested important areas for research. These findings were supported and extended in a 1987 conference cosponsored by the National Institutes of Health and the National Osteoporosis Foundation.

The public is finally becoming aware of osteoporosis. Why, then, have we written this book? *First,* researchers have discovered much more about osteoporosis—its causes, who is and who is not likely to develop it, and how it can be prevented. *Second,* there are new ways of measuring the amount of bone tissue—sophisticated X-ray methods that will soon be available to almost everyone, though not everyone will need to make use of them. *Third,* myths have arisen that demand careful clarification. It is a myth, for example, that estrogen therapy commonly causes cancer. It is likewise a myth that calcium is a cure-all for osteoporosis or that calcium is not important in preventing osteoporosis. You, our readers, should know what is and what is not known about this condition, and what new knowledge is on the horizon. Health awareness has increased. Fitness and nutrition are topical, and a "smokeless society" is being discussed.

Striving for better health is a top priority for everyone. You should not sit back and wait for the inevitability of bone loss. Prevention of osteoporosis and of the fractures it causes requires your participation, commitment, and knowledge.

1 • Understanding Osteoporosis— An Overview

You may have seen at some time a hunchbacked elderly woman struggling to climb stairs or board a bus—as if she bore the weight of the world. Osteoporosis is very likely the condition that crippled that woman and jeopardized a most precious commodity, her independence.

Osteoporosis has affected her vertebrae, the building blocks of her spine. Weakened by the loss of bone tissue, they were gradually crushed by the weight of her body (even though she may be far from heavy), shrinking and deforming her.

Bones are hard structures that support and protect the body and store the body's calcium. How is it that the vertebrae—or, for that matter, the hip and many other bones—become so fragile? Simply because their strength depends on the amount and nature of the tissue within them.

BONE AS LIVING TISSUE

Unlike the steel superstructure of a building, bone is living tissue that renews itself continuously. This renewal process, called remodeling, enables bones to repair themselves and to release calcium into the bloodstream. In this way, bones compensate for any dietary inadequacy of calcium, ensuring the normal levels of blood calcium required for organs such as the brain, kidneys, and the heart to work properly. Remodeling involves tearing down and rebuilding, both going on at several million places throughout the skeleton.

Bones lengthen and widen during growth and continue to thicken even after growth stops. As a result, bones are heaviest and strongest between the ages of twenty-five and forty—when the skeleton matures. After bones have fully matured, they begin to waste away. Slowly and silently, tissue is lost from within, progressively thinning the walls and framework. Losses continue until sometime in the eighties. Some people already have thin bones at maturity; some lose too much bone thereafter. In both cases, the end result may be the same—too little bone tissue, or osteoporosis. Women have smaller, thinner bones than men, and they lose bone rapidly during the five to ten years that follow the menopause (change of life). Small wonder that osteoporosis is more common in women than in men.

NORMAL BONE AND BONE WITH OSTEOPOROSIS

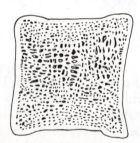

Normal Vertebra

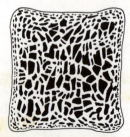

Vertebra with Osteoporosis

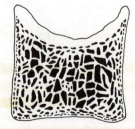

Crushed Vertebra with Osteoporosis

FRACTURE

Osteoporosis is not really a disease; it causes no symptoms. It does not "cause" a fracture. What it does is increase the likelihood of fracture, the chances of breaking a bone. A woman with osteoporosis can crush a vertebra merely by lifting a lightweight bag of groceries out of a car trunk. But not everyone with osteoporosis will suffer a fracture. There are an estimated 25 million people in the United States with osteoporosis—including one-third to one-half of postmenopausal women and nearly one-half of all people over the age of seventy-five. Although most will never break a bone, they are much more likely to do so than people without osteoporosis. And if they do, the consequences can be devastating. Of the nearly quarter of a million people with osteoporosis who break a hip each year, nearly half will never be able to live independently, one-quarter will require nursing home care, and as many as 10 percent will die within one year because of diseases associated with immobility—blood clots on the lungs, pneumonia, and malnutrition.

RISK FACTORS

Who will develop osteoporosis and who already has it are key questions that will be addressed in later chapters. Both questions deal with the issue of risk, or likelihood, of developing the condition. Everyone has *some* risk, ranging from very low to very high. Almost all high-risk people are likely to develop osteoporosis; at the other end of the spectrum, almost no one at low risk need be concerned. Many factors contribute to overall risk for a disorder as complicated as osteoporosis—age, sex, race, heredity, and so-called lifestyle factors such as diet, exercise, smoking, and taking certain prescription drugs.

Why be concerned about risk? Because osteoporosis *can* be prevented and risk *reduced*, not only by changes in lifestyle but also with medications. Adequate calcium nutrition and exercise are important, as are avoidance of cigarette smoking and alcohol abuse. Estrogen therapy has been proven to diminish bone loss in postmenopausal women. Many individuals, unless confronted with the fact that they are at high risk, will simply not make necessary lifestyle changes. And medications are not for everyone. Some women are not candidates for or won't accept estrogen therapy, and, since estrogen fosters female sex traits, men are ineligible. Calcitonin is an alternate form of treatment but is expensive, must be injected like insulin, and has not been tested as thoroughly as estrogen. A reasonable approach is for individuals to know first what their risk is and then work to reduce that risk, if it is high, through lifestyle changes, medications, or both.

TECHNIQUES TO MEASURE BONE MASS

The key to healthy bones is bone mass, or density, scientific terms that describe the amount of hard bone tissue one has and therefore how strong the bones are. In deciding who is and who isn't at high risk for osteoporosis, two factors must be considered: (1) how much bone tissue is there, especially in the fracture-prone bones such as the vertebrae and the hip bone, and (2) how fast the bone tissue is disappearing with advancing age. Fortunately, bone mass can now be measured reliably, using techniques that are more sophisticated and sensitive than X-ray methods applied to the spine, hip, and other bones. The techniques can't be used with everyone; they're still too expensive to be routinely done, considering the many people who do not need them. But they do help confirm the assessment of risk in likely candidates for osteoporosis, discover whether recommended preventive approaches are working, and aid in diagnosing osteoporosis in patients who have broken a bone. They are valuable research aids, too, since they enable scientists to study the effects of an agent on bone loss. Improvements now on the horizon are likely to increase the effectiveness of these techniques. Also under development are new ways of diagnosing fast bone loss—chemical tests performed on the blood and urine that give valuable information—since it is the "fast bone loser" who may be at highest risk for osteoporosis.

PREVENTION

It is not enough to learn about the nature of bone, how bone is lost, and who is and is not likely to develop osteoporosis. What readers should know is how to prevent it, and, for those already afflicted, how to live with it. Among the preventive strategies are calcium, exercise, and estrogen therapy.

The role of calcium in preventing osteoporosis has been controversial. Advertisements have proclaimed calcium as a cure-all for the condition despite conflicting scientific studies. The reader should know these important facts about calcium: (1) Everybody must consume calcium. If one avoids calcium for a long time (months to years), the skeleton becomes brittle or soft. (2) Calcium needs vary greatly from person to person and, in the same person, at different life stages. For example, adolescents, pregnant women, and many elderly people need more calcium than healthy, nonpregnant younger adults. (3) Without extensive laboratory tests, too elaborate for routine care, physicians cannot determine exactly what an individual's needs are. (4) Our recommendations are meant to accommodate most people's calcium requirement without causing side effects. (5) Women should know that calcium will not substitute for estrogen treatment as a way to diminish the rapid loss of bone tissue that follows the menopause. But there is evidence that calcium does help and that estrogen therapy is more beneficial when one's calcium intake is adequate. (6) Certain calcium supplements are reasonable substitutes for calcium in milk and other dietary sources. Not all supplements provide bioavailable calcium—calcium that is easily dissolved in the stomach and absorbed into the body. The reader will learn answers to questions about calcium such as, How much calcium is needed each day? What are the food sources of calcium? Which calcium supplements have been tested for bioavailability, and how should supplements be used? How much calcium is too much? Is calcium really good for high blood pressure, and does it prevent cancer? Who should avoid calcium supplements? What should the children and grandchildren be told about calcium?

Recent scientific evidence points to physical exercise as beneficial to the skeleton. Certainly the health benefits of exercise are well known: weight loss, a trim figure, improved muscle tone, and reduced risk of heart disease. Now it appears that certain kinds of exercise help build bone during growth and maturation and may diminish aging-associated bone loss. The reader will learn about the best exercises for the skeleton—what kind, how often, and for how long—and what precautions should be taken when starting a program.

The female hormone estrogen is needed for reproduction, vaginal health, and breast development. It also protects the skeleton. At menopause, a woman's ovaries are making too little estrogen for any of these purposes. In addition to physical disturbances, such as hot flushes and sweats, there is a dramatic speeding up of bone loss, lasting for at least five to ten years. It is not surprising, therefore, that taking estrogen pills can prevent the disturbing symptoms of menopause *and* diminish bone loss. In fact, the Food and Drug Administration (FDA), the government agency that approves new drugs for marketing in the United States, has approved oral estrogen pills to treat osteoporosis. Although reasonably safe when properly used and widely accepted in recent years, estrogen therapy does have side effects. When recommended to prevent osteoporosis, it is prescribed only for women who are at risk. In fact, progesterone, another female hormone, when prescribed with estrogen, helps prevent the most important complication of estrogen therapy, cancer of the endometrium (lining of the uterus, or womb). The reader must consider several key issues: Who should consider estrogen therapy? Who must avoid estrogen? What are its complications, and how can they be avoided? What preparations and doses are most effective? How long should treatment last, and what happens to bone when treatment is stopped? Does estrogen prevent heart disease?

LIVING WITH THE CONDITION

Since estrogen therapy works but is not for all women or any men, and since calcium and exercise in themselves may not be completely protective, the reader should know about other treatment options, both available (such as calcitonin) and on the horizon. But what about the many individuals who already have osteoporosis? It may be possible to block further bone loss, and new ways to rebuild bones are being tested. People with severe osteoporosis can live with their condition; afflicted readers can learn to avoid the situations and hazards that can cause a brittle bone to break. An older person who does not fall is unlikely to suffer a hip fracture and will almost certainly not break a wrist bone. The reader needs to understand falling, since changes in lifestyle and environment can prevent the fall that triggers this most serious of skeletal injuries.

CURRENT RESEARCH

Medical research is a promise—society's investment in the future—and osteoporosis, now recognized as a major public health problem, is receiving increased scientific attention (though, in overview, not nearly enough). It is important to become educated about the most exciting current research—what the next five to ten years will bring. There is every reason to hope that osteoporosis can be eliminated within the next twenty-five years, with proper attention to research.

OSTEOPOROSIS: VITAL STATISTICS

- Afflicts 25 million Americans, including one-third to one-half of postmenopausal women and nearly half of all people over age seventy-five.
- Causes 1.3 million fractures annually, including nearly 250,000 hip fractures.
- Costs an estimated 10 billion dollars each year.

2 • Form and Function of Bones

Most advanced life forms have extremely strong inner skeletons—unlike primitive species, which have an outside skeleton or none at all. We take for granted the benefits of our skeleton—protection, support, anchorage of muscles, leverage, and storage of the vital mineral calcium. Our skeleton is a truly remarkable organ. Imagine what life would be like without it!

WHAT BONES ARE MADE OF

To work, bones must be strong and hard. They receive strength and hardness from two kinds of chemicals—proteins and minerals. The leathery protein collagen is the supportive framework of virtually all tissues in the body; hence, it is known as one of the connective tissues. Bone collagen is special, for unlike collagen in other tissues, it is a magnet for the calcium-containing mineral that makes bone hard. Calcium in bone combines with other elements—including phosphorus, oxygen, and hydrogen—to form crystals much like the crystals of sodium chloride, ordinary table salt. Bone crystal is known as hydroxyapatite. Bone collagen also attracts other elements; in fact, bone is a waste storage depot for some toxic elements, including lead and mercury. In addition, bone

UPPER PART OF FEMUR, OR HIP BONE

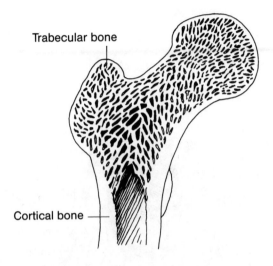

takes up and holds, or binds, fluoride—the same fluoride that many communities add to their water supply to prevent dental cavities—and fluoride in pill form is now being studied as a way of treating osteoporosis. Strontium is another element attracted to bone. Anthropologists and archaeologists learn about the feeding habits of ancient animals and humans by measuring the amount of strontium in excavated bones. Meat-eaters accumulate less strontium than vegetable-eaters. Radioactive strontium, a major part of fallout from nuclear tests and accidents, is harmful because it reaches bone and stays there a long time.

DESIGN OF SKELETON

The remarkable strength and hardness of bone tissue does not guarantee good function. It is because of the ingenious way the 206 bones in the human body are designed—the distribution and shape of bone tissue—that bones func-

THE SKELETAL SYSTEM

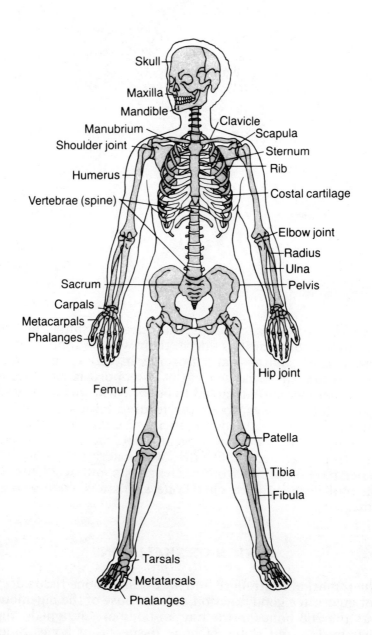

tion so well. Bone tissue is arranged two different ways: in 80 percent of the skeleton, it is densely packed in layers called compact, or cortical, bone, generally forming a tough outer shell, or cortex; and in 20 percent, it is arrayed in a meshwork of thin, tough, bony plates (trabecular, or cancellous, bone—also called spongy bone because it is porous), filling cavities within the bones. These cavities also contain bone marrow, the blood cell-producing tissue, and fat. The cortex is the thickest, densest, and strongest part of bone. It receives added strength because its tissue consists of many tightly packed rods, called haversian systems, firmly glued together with a natural adhesive substance. Each rod contains a blood vessel that carries nutrients to and waste products away from bone tissue. Trabecular bone tissue exchanges nutrients and waste products with the bone marrow that surrounds it.

Bones are functional in design. Protective bones such as the skull and pelvis are thick and dense. Arm and leg bones, by contrast, are long, hollowed-out cylinders, combining strength and lightness. Engineers recognize the cylinder as the geometric form best able to withstand forces from above and below (compression), as well as bending and twisting forces (torsion). Imagine the pressures your leg bones endure without breaking when you run and jump. The haversian systems in the cortex of these bones run lengthwise, thus adding to their strength. Resiliency characterizes the bones of the spine (vertebrae). These twenty-four cubelike building blocks are filled with spongy, or trabecular, bone capable of cushioning the forces of upright posture. In forming a spinal pillar, individual vertebrae are separated by soft pads (intervertebral discs), providing an added cushioning effect and the flexibility needed for bending and twisting. (Normally, those discs are held in place by connective tissue collars. Occasionally, a collar breaks, allowing the softer disc material to escape from the spaces between the vertebrae and press on nearby nerves, causing severe pain, weakness, or numbness. This is the so-called slipped, or ruptured, disc, which must be treated by bed rest, surgery, or the injection of an enzyme that digests the escaped disc material.)

Joints connecting bones together complete the skeleton's functional design. Some joints, such as those of the knee and hip, permit a wide range of motion yet can support heavy weight. In these movable joints, the adjacent ends of the bones are capped by cartilage tissue and separated by a pouch filled with an oily lubricant, joint fluid. Hence, joint motion is smooth. Other joints, such as those that connect the pelvis to the upper part of the tailbone (sacroiliac joints) are strong but relatively inflexible. (Like bone tissue, joint cartilage may wear away with advancing age, though the process by which this occurs is different from that in bone. The condition is called osteoarthritis. It is a major cause of pain, stiffness, and immobility.)

FRACTURE AND IMMOBILITY

Remarkably, healthy bones do not break except under the most extraordinary circumstances. They tolerate enormous forces. But breaking a major bone causes virtually immediate immobilization followed by a long period of healing and convalescence. Loss of independence and freedom are all-too-frequent results. Osteoporosis means that even a seemingly trivial injury can produce a fracture. And the consequences of immobility are more severe in older people, the very ones who are, of course, most likely to have osteoporosis and break bones. Preventing osteoporosis and the fractures it causes is one way to remain independent and free.

THE FUNCTIONS OF BONE

- Protects vital organs.
- Supports and shapes the body and its parts.
- Anchors muscles and provides leverage.
- Stores calcium and other minerals.

---

3 • Fracture—A Hazard of Osteoporosis

Osteoporosis, the silent thief, has only one immediate complication—fracture. A fracture is a breach, or break, in the normal surface, or contour, of bone tissue. Different bones break in different ways, depending on their shape and the way they are injured. For example, weakened vertebrae, building blocks of the spine, are compressed, collapsed, or crushed by the body's weight. Bones of the arms and legs, cylindrical or tubular in structure, may break when bent or twisted. Fractures may cause symptoms: pain, a limb that cannot be used, numbness, paralysis, protrusion of a broken bone through the skin (compound fracture), and bleeding. Or, they may produce deformity that is so slight or gradual as to go unnoticed. Although the presence of osteoporosis increases one's chances of breaking almost any bone, fractures of the spine, hip, and wrist are most common.

SPINAL FRACTURES

Spinal fractures are most likely to complicate osteoporosis between the ages of fifty-five and seventy-five and usually occur in women as a consequence of rapid loss of bone tissue from the vertebrae after menopause. In fact, women are seven times more likely to suffer a spinal

PRINCIPAL SITES OF FRACTURES

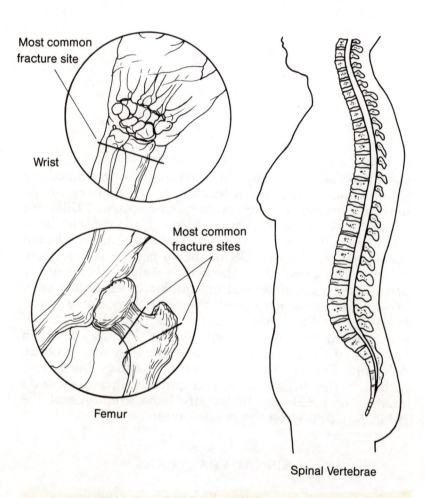

fracture than men. X rays will show fracture of the spine in many women aged seventy or over.

Vertebrae collapse, or cave in, when they fracture. The collapse, or compression, may be sudden, the entire vertebra crushed completely almost in an instant, or it may be gradual, occurring over many months to years as different portions of the bone give way in stages. Collapsed vertebrae do not "heal" by rebuilding themselves—they remain collapsed forever. Microscopic inspection of vertebrae weakened by osteoporosis shows that many individual trabeculae, tiny plates of bone within the vertebrae, fracture (microfractures) before the entire bone gives way. Lifting, twisting, sitting down hard, and arising from bed quickly are actions that may trigger a compression fracture. Complete compressions are often painful; a sudden attack of severe pain in the middle of the back worsened by strains such as coughing, bearing down, deep breathing, and any motion is most typical. The pain can last for days and even weeks. Rarely, a completely collapsed vertebra can press on the spinal cord, the core of nerve tissue that transmits nerve impulses between the brain and other parts of the body, or on the nerves that pass to the body from the spinal cord. When this happens, numbness, pain radiating down a leg, or paralysis can occur.

Diagnosis of Spinal Fracture

Many conditions can produce the same symptoms as a spinal fracture—severe back muscle strain, a slipped disc, bleeding around the spine, spinal infections or arthritis, or diseases of the internal organs and tissues near the spine (the kidneys, the aorta, and the pancreas, to name a few). Consequently, diagnosis is important. Examination of the back may reveal tenderness over the crushed vertebra or the nearby muscles, and an X ray will show the collapse. Rest and painkilling medicine are the best treatments. Application of mild heat and brief traction to the back may help relieve the painful muscle spasms that accompany the fracture.

Most collapse fractures produce no pain or pain that is so slight and transient that it is not thought to be serious. Indeed, women may have painless fractures with-

COLLAPSED VERTEBRAE

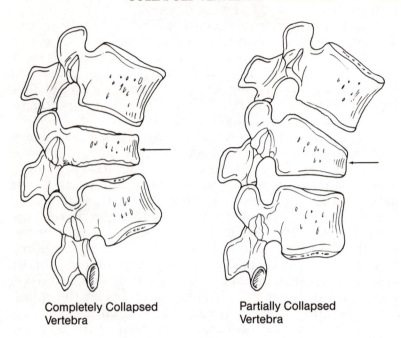

Completely Collapsed Vertebra

Partially Collapsed Vertebra

out seeking medical attention until they become concerned by their loss of height and the development of a hunched back.

Deformity from Spinal Fracture

Collapse of individual vertebra leads to shrinkage; a woman who has collapsed seven or eight vertebrae, an all-too-common occurrence, may lose four to six inches in height. Furthermore, the vertebrae of the upper spine often collapse to a greater degree in the front than in the back and become wedge-shaped. Thus, the upper spine bends forward, causing the back to hunch over. The chest is shortened, and often the bottom ribs rest upon the bones of the pelvis. The abdomen, also compressed, bulges, and digestion of food may be compromised. Occasionally, the chest is so shrunken that breathing is difficult, and pneumonia becomes a danger. Over a third of the women with collapsed vertebrae also develop a curvature of the lower spine. The deformity caused by multiple collapse fractures may in itself cause pain and stiffness, turning many commonplace movements into difficult chores at best and impossibilities at worst. Use of a soft abdominal corset (not a rigid one, which can impair breathing), special exercises prescribed by a physiatrist (a specialist in rehabilitation) or physical therapist, and a program of movement reeducation (how to move without incurring further injury, stiffness, or pain) may help maximize mobility and minimize stiffness. Clearly, however, collapse of vertebrae is a condition to avoid.

HIP FRACTURES

Hip fracture can be a major tragedy in an older person's life. It is actually a broken thighbone (femur) that is known as a broken hip. The femur normally bends inward toward the body at its upper end, joining the pelvis like a ball in a socket. It is the angled upper portion of the femur where most hip fractures occur. They tend to happen at an older age than spinal fractures and are only twice as likely

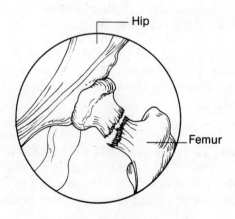

HIP FRACTURE

to affect women as men, in contrast to the very high proportion of women sustaining collapse fractures of the vertebrae. There are two reasons hip fracture is likely in both men and women. First, weakening of the hip bone, or proximal femur (thighbone), requires the loss of cortical bone—which is a more gradual consequence of aging than is loss of trabecular bone—and almost anyone who lives long enough can suffer sufficient cortical bone loss to jeopardize the hip. Second, a hip does not often break spontaneously; an injury, usually a fall, almost always causes the fracture. And the elderly, men and women alike, are much more likely to fall than the young. This combination—osteoporosis in the hip and a fall—is all too common in the lives of the aged.

Hip fracture in elderly people can cause suffering and even death. It almost always produces severe pain and immobility. Many but not all afflicted patients will undergo some kind of surgery. Bone tissue has amazing self-healing power—it is the only tissue that can heal without a scar, though mending is slow, often taking many months. One exception is the part of the femur that usually breaks. Whether or not osteoporosis is present, a pin is inserted to aid healing, or a prosthesis is inserted to create "instant" healing. A prolonged, painful period of rehabilitation may follow. About one in five elderly patients will not live more than two years after the fracture. It is not the broken bone itself that is so serious but rather the complications that can be caused by being bedridden, or nearly so—pneumonia, blood clots traveling to the lungs, depression, malnutrition, bladder infections, and bed sores. Nearly half of elderly patients who were living independent lives will never be able to do so after the fracture, and one in four will need to be in a skilled nursing facility for a long time. Many hip fractures can be prevented by reducing bone loss and decreasing the chances of falling.

WRIST AND OTHER FRACTURES

Although spinal and hip fractures are the most devastating complications of osteoporosis, severe bone loss makes almost any bone brittle and susceptible to fracture; particularly common are fractures of the bones of the wrist and upper arm, the ribs, and the pelvis. Seemingly trivial injury is often all that is needed to break these bones. While most fractures will cause at least some discomfort, more severe fractures can be fatal. The key is to prevent osteoporosis and, if it is already present, to learn to live with the disorder, chiefly by avoiding injuries such as falls.

THE MAIN FRACTURES OF OSTEOPOROSIS

Spinal Fractures (Collapse, or Crush, Fractures of Vertebrae)
- Estimated to be present in 5 million American women.
- Found in over one-third of women over the age of sixty-five.
- 7 times more common in women than in men.
- Fifty-five- to seventy-five-year-old women at greatest risk.
- A major cause of pain, debility, height loss, and deformity.

Hip Fractures
- Nearly 250,000 each year in the United States.
- 2 times more common in women than in men.
- 1 in 12 thirty-five-year-old women can expect to suffer a hip fracture in later years.
- 1 in 5 victims will not survive more than two years afterward.
- 1 in 4 victims will enter a skilled nursing facility.
- Nearly one-half of all victims will not live independently again.
- Sixty-five- to eighty-five-year-old people at greatest risk.
- Often caused by falls inside the home.

Wrist Fractures
- As frequent as hip fractures.
- 6 times more common in women than in men.
- Usually caused by falls outside the home.

---

4 • Bone Changes with Age

Bones are constantly changing. They grow longer and wider during fetal life, infancy, childhood, and adolescence. Specialized growth centers, called epiphyses, add new tissue to the ends of the bones. Growth centers stop working by late adolescence, when maximum height is reached. A thin layer of tissue covering the outer surfaces of bone, the periosteum, also generates new bone tissue. As a result, bones slowly widen.

REMODELING

Bones also change by a continuous process of self-renewal, or remodeling. This process is so vigorous that it can replace an entire bone in five years. At millions of places throughout the skeleton, a small amount of bone tissue is removed (bone resorption) and then replaced with new tissue (bone formation) that is indistinguishable from the old. Remodeling at each location begins when a team of bone cells (osteoclasts) erodes into the bone surface, dissolving bone tissue along the way. Calcium dissolved in the process passes into the bloodstream. After a certain amount of tissue has been resorbed, a different team of bone cells (osteoblasts) migrates into the eroded area and fills it in with new bone tissue. The entire process, from initiation of resorption to completion of repair, takes about 100 days. Remodeling is painless; it occurs mainly on the internal surfaces of each bone. Normally, the balance between resorption and formation determines whether bone tissue accumulates or disappears. During the growing and maturing years, more bone is formed than is resorbed. After about age thirty to thirty-five for trabecular bones such as the vertebrae (spine), and age forty-five to fifty for compact bones such as the femur (thighbone), formation lags behind resorption, and bone is lost. Slow, gradual losses continue into the late eighties, reflecting the buildup of slight imbalances at each remodeling location. So it is that, with advancing age, constant remodeling jeopardizes the skeleton. Everyone loses bone tissue as a part of aging, regardless of sex, lifestyle, or race. Osteoporosis is present when there is too little bone tissue, making the bones brittle and apt to fracture. Not building enough bone in the first place, or losing too much later on, causes this condition.

Remodeling does not exist merely to renew the skeleton. It allows bone to act as a storehouse for calcium. One of the major functions of remodeling is to release from bone some of its enormous calcium reserve when the body is deprived of calcium.

REMODELING

1. Resting Phase

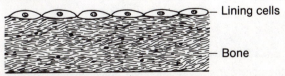

A bone surface is covered by a protective layer of bone cells—called lining cells.

---

2. Resorption

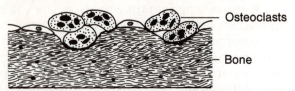

During resorption, osteoclasts (large cells with many nuclei) invade the bone surface and erode it, dissolving the mineral and the matrix.

3. Resorption Complete

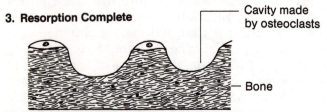

A small cavity is created in the bone surface—resorption complete.

4. Formation—Repair

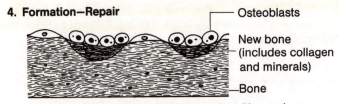

Bone-forming cells begin to fill in the cavity with new bone.

5. Repair Complete

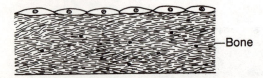

Finally, the bone surface is completely restored.

THE SKELETON AS A STOREHOUSE FOR CALCIUM

All organs need calcium to work properly. It is calcium in the bloodstream that energizes the countless electrical impulses and chemical reactions that operate the brain, heart, and other tissues. Dangerously low levels of calcium cause organ malfunction; life-threatening seizures and abnormalities in the heartbeat are the most serious results.

Foods and dietary supplements are the body's *only* outside sources of calcium. The only natural way to gain calcium is to consume it (calcium can be supplied intravenously in emergency situations). To be useful, calcium that is consumed must be transported from the stomach and intestines into the bloodstream—this is known as calcium absorption. Calcium is eliminated from the body in two main ways. Unabsorbed calcium left in the intestine, a surprisingly high one-half to three-quarters of the amount consumed, appears in the stool. The kidneys eliminate calcium from the body by adding it to urine.

Calcium must be consumed and absorbed to satisfy the needs of the body, and elimination, mainly in the urine, continues even when it is not. Thus, serious calcium deficits can result from prolonged deficiencies in supply.

A ready supply of calcium in the skeleton comes into play when too little calcium is consumed or absorbed or when too much is wasted. Bones contain about 99 percent of the 1,000 grams of calcium in the average human body, a substantial reservoir indeed. Calcium is leeched from bone when needed; a decrease in blood calcium triggers bone resorption—mobilizing calcium into the bloodstream and preventing organ malfunction. Calcium is not withdrawn from bony stores without a high cost; that cost is the loss of bone tissue and, therefore, of bone strength.

The calcium reservoir is so large that it can easily withstand small, short-term withdrawals. In fact, even months of dietary calcium deficiency can be tolerated without jeopardizing the skeleton. An insufficient intake of calcium for years, however, as is *common* in the U.S. population, can place the skeleton in jeopardy. Bone loss also accompanies medical conditions in which calcium is not well absorbed or is eliminated excessively in the urine. Deficiency of calcium is particularly dangerous in growing children and adolescents, whose bones need to *gain* calcium, and in individuals over the age of forty-five, who are already losing bone tissue because of the aging process. Remember, osteoporosis comes from inadequate accumulation of bone tissue during growth and maturation *and* excessive losses thereafter.

Although bone is the only calcium storehouse, it is not the only organ that works to prevent calcium deficiency; normally, the intestine and the kidneys also help. When the level of calcium in blood falls, the intestine normally absorbs more of the calcium in the diet and the kidneys eliminate less. The bones, intestine, and kidneys do not act spontaneously—they are directed by chemical messengers. Ensuring that there is enough calcium in the blood is the task of a sophisticated chemical control circuit. First, biological sensors monitor blood calcium. Second, detecting low levels, they signal specialized internal glands to inject a corrective hormone (chemical messenger), parathyroid hormone, into the bloodstream. Third, this hormone stimulates bone resorption, which inserts more calcium into the blood. Parathyroid hormone restores blood calcium in two more ways: it reduces calcium elimination in the urine, and it brings about an increase in calcium absorption from the intestine. (Diverse hormones control virtually all bodily functions. Calcium regulators are but one example; another is insulin. Released by the pancreas in response to a rise in blood sugar, after a meal, insulin signals muscle and other tissues to burn the sugar. Lack of insulin, diabetes mellitus, blocks this process.) Fourth, hormone production stops when blood calcium is restored to normal.

Parathyroid Hormone, Calcitonin, and Vitamin D

Parathyroid hormone, the main line of defense against a low blood calcium level, is normally secreted by four tiny glands (parathyroid glands) situated behind the thyroid gland, just below the Adam's apple. It is the key that unlocks the calcium storehouse in bone.

HORMONES THAT REGULATE BLOOD CALCIUM

Parathyroid Hormone
- Made by small glands in the neck.
- Activated by low blood calcium.
- Stimulates bone resorption—increases release of calcium from bone stores.
- Acts on kidneys to—
    reduce calcium loss in urine.
    convert vitamin D to an active chemical form of the vitamin, thereby stimulating absorption of dietary calcium.

Calcitonin
- Made by thyroid gland.
- Activated by high blood calcium.
- Blocks bone resorption—reduces release of calcium from bone stores.

Vitamin D
- Not strictly a vitamin, since it is made in the skin cells during exposure to ultraviolet rays.
- Must be converted to an active chemical form of the vitamin by liver and kidneys before it works.
- Stimulates calcium absorption from the intestine.

Two other substances, calcitonin and vitamin D, participate in calcium regulation. Calcitonin, a hormone made by specialized cells in the thyroid gland itself, blocks bone remodeling when blood calcium levels are elevated, counteracting the effect of parathyroid hormone. Synthetic calcitonin is now used to treat patients with osteoporosis (see chapter 12).

Vitamin D stimulates the intestinal absorption of calcium (and other elements, such as phosphorus and magnesium).

A vitamin is a chemical compound that controls vital processes but cannot be made by the body; it is an essential component of the diet. Vitamin D is essential, but since it is also made in skin tissue during exposure to ultraviolet rays of the sun (hence the term *sunshine vi-*

tamin), it is not strictly speaking a vitamin. Vitamin D, whether consumed in foods or vitamin supplements or made by skin, is not active; it must be chemically converted in the body by the liver and kidneys to an active form called by the scientifically precise term *1,25 vitamin D*. Vitamin D in the 1,25 form is the substance that actually stimulates intestinal calcium absorption. One of the ways in which parathyroid hormone works to protect against a low blood calcium level is to increase the activation of vitamin D by the kidneys. Lack of sunlight exposure; dietary deficiency; and disease of the kidneys, liver, or intestines produce vitamin D (hence 1,25) deficiency. This condition leads to too little magnesium and phosphorus in the blood and insufficient calcium for bone growth. Soft bones may result, a disease known as rickets in children and osteomalacia in adults. Too much vitamin D (often caused by taking excessive vitamin supplements) can cause severe, sometimes fatal, elevations in blood calcium and kidney stones. Too much vitamin D masquerades as parathyroid hormone, stimulating the loss of bone tissue.

The living, responsive nature of bone tissue—functioning as a calcium storehouse—makes osteoporosis possible. Scientific discovery of the complexities of calcium metabolism has provided crucial clues to the nature of osteoporosis and approaches to its prevention and treatment.

Thyroid Hormone and Growth Hormone

Other hormones not involved in regulating blood calcium nevertheless play important roles in bone growth and remodeling, therefore influencing the amount of bone tissue in the body. These include thyroid hormone and growth hormone.

Thyroid hormone is made by the thyroid gland, located in the neck below the Adam's apple. This hormone determines how fast tissues grow and burn sugar, fats, and proteins. Thyroid hormone exists in two iodine-containing forms, thyroxine (T_4) and triiodothyronine (T_3); T_4 contains more iodine. Thyroid hormone speeds up bone remodeling; bone loss can result from an overactive thyroid gland or from taking too much thyroid hormone in pill form.

As its name implies, growth hormone stimulates the growth of the body and virtually all of its tissues, including the bones. Growth hormone is produced by the pituitary gland, a small organ at the base of the brain. Its main action is to prompt the liver and other organs to make a second growth hormone called somatomedin, which actually conveys the growth hormone message to the rest of the body; it is responsible for the actions of growth hormone. Somatomedin stimulates bone growth; evidence indicates that less somatomedin is produced with advancing age—a decline that may contribute to aging-associated loss of bone tissue.

Sex Hormones

Sex hormones are so named because they are needed for reproduction and sexual development. Estrogen and progesterone are the main female sex hormones; they are made in the ovaries. Testosterone is the principal male sex hormone; it is made by the testicles beginning at puberty, when the testicles become capable of producing sperm cells. In both sexes, the adrenal glands, located above the kidneys, also produce female and male sex hormones, but in much smaller amounts than the ovaries and the testicles. Fat tissue and muscles can make a little estrogen as well. Women who are obese or muscular have higher es-

---

OTHER HORMONES THAT INFLUENCE BONE REMODELING

Thyroid Hormone
Growth Hormone
Somatomedin
"Sex" Hormones–Estrogen, Progesterone, and Testosterone
Cortisone (see chapter 5)
Prolactin (see chapter 5)

trogen levels in their blood than those who are lean. Estrogen tends to block the resorption phase of bone remodeling; consequently, a diminished estrogen supply leads to excessive bone loss. Progesterone and testosterone may have similar effects on bone, and, unlike estrogens, may also be able to stimulate bone formation. But clearly, estrogen is the main protective hormone for bones in women; testosterone serves that function in men.

The ovaries' major tasks are to release mature eggs (ova), a process known as ovulation, and to make estrogen and progesterone. These hormones serve multiple purposes—they are needed for ovulation, for initiating pregnancy, for normal lubrication of the vagina, and for normal breast development. Other hormones are needed to prepare the breasts for lactation, or milk production, including prolactin, a pituitary hormone, and a milk-producing hormone made in the placenta. The ovaries do not work automatically; they are controlled by hormones from the pituitary gland, which, in turn, is regulated by the brain.

The Menstrual Cycle

The menstrual cycle is a complex series of monthly events that prepare the endometrium (lining of the uterus, or womb) to receive and nurture a fertilized ovum and include shedding of the endometrium as waste tissue (menstruation) if the ovum is not fertilized. From birth, ovaries are endowed with a rich supply of follicles—structures that give rise to mature ova. One of these follicles will usually yield an ovum during each normal menstrual cycle.

The follicle-enriched ovaries are first stimulated into activity by pituitary hormones during puberty, usually at a little over twelve and a half years of age. Ovarian maturation results in the first menstrual period, known as menarche. During the menopausal years, some thirty-five to forty years later, the ovaries lose their ability to produce ova, and their synthesis of female hormones declines dramatically. Between menarche and menopause, a woman will have hundreds of menstrual cycles; only pregnancy or medical conditions will interrupt these cycles.

A normal menstrual cycle, lasting about twenty-eight days, begins with the onset of menstrual bleeding (or period). It is during the four to five days of bleeding that the ovaries, directed by the pituitary gland, begin to make increasing amounts of estrogen. After menstruation stops, estrogen acts to thicken the endometrium. At the same time, an ovum is maturing within an ovary. About thirteen to fourteen days from the start of the period, an ovum leaves the ovary and passes into an adjacent tube (fallopian tube), where it can be fertilized if sperm are present. If so, the ovary begins to make large amounts of progesterone, which softens the thickened endometrium and increases its supply of tiny blood vessels—all in preparation for implantation, a process whereby a fertilized ovum attaches to and buries itself in the endometrium and begins to develop into a fetus. The ovaries are then shut off, and the placenta, a newly developed mass of special tissue that feeds the fetus and removes its waste products, becomes the supplier of female sex hormones for the duration of the pregnancy. Without fertilization, progesterone production declines. Fifteen to sixteen days after ovulation, the endometrium is shed, and menstrual bleeding again ensues.

The Menopause

The climacteric, or change of life, is the period in a woman's life when her ovaries become inactive—ovulation ceases and hormone production wanes. Normally, it is gradual, extending over many years, and is often heralded by irregular menstrual periods or increased menstrual bleeding. The menopause actually starts with a woman's final menstrual period. This last episode of menstruation, usually occurring at about age fifty-one, signals the menopause. Physicians diagnose the menopause when a woman has had no menstrual period for at least six months and when blood tests disclose the virtual cessation of ovarian hormone production. Infertility and reduction in female sex hormones are the consequences of menopause. Lowered amounts of estrogen cause a number of disturbances, speed up the loss of bone tissue, and may set the stage for an increased incidence of heart disease.

(Estrogen protects women not only against bone loss but may also protect against atherosclerosis—narrowing and clogging of the arteries with cholesterol-filled plaques, a process that sets the stage for most heart attacks.)

Menopause is a part of the normal aging process. All women who live long enough will experience it. Natural menopause may occur prematurely, before the age of forty-five, or can be delayed until the mid-fifties. Menopause also results from surgical removal of both ovaries (bilateral oophorectomy), often performed at the time of a hysterectomy (removal of the uterus), from damage to ovaries caused by X-ray or chemical treatments for cancer, and from various diseases that can destroy the ovaries. Unlike natural menopause, menopause following oophorectomy is abrupt, and estrogen production falls quickly to very low levels. The adrenal glands continue to make small amounts of estrogen, as do fat and muscle tissues. For all practical purposes, however, bilateral oophorectomy causes severe deficiency of estrogen. Chapter 11 describes how estrogen treatment is used to control the disturbing symptoms of menopause, reduce the loss of bone tissue, and possibly protect against heart disease.

Decline in Testosterone Production

The production of testosterone, the male sex hormone, does not exhibit the kinds of cycles that characterize estrogen and progesterone production in women. Although less testosterone is made later in life, the decline is not as abrupt as is the decline in estrogen production in women and usually does not begin until about age seventy. Thus, men do not experience anything like the female menopause. Their reproductive ability and sexual potency, determined in part by testosterone, wanes with advancing age; but men can maintain normal sexual activity, though they usually can no longer reproduce, into their eighties. The absence of "menopause" means that men in their fifties do not lose bone tissue rapidly, unlike postmenopausal women. Whether reductions in testosterone contribute to the gradual aging-associated bone loss experienced by all men is uncertain.

5 • Risk Factors—and Protective Factors— for Osteoporosis

Osteoporosis is, for many people, a preventable condition. Loss of bone tissue can be reduced; there are not yet safe methods for restoring bone tissue, though several now being tested offer promise. Some preventive approaches, such as regular weight-bearing exercise, can be recommended widely, even though their value has not been established through rigid scientific testing, because they seem to be helpful to many and are generally safe and cheap. More effective strategies, such as the prescription of certain hormones, must be reserved for individuals at special risk, since these strategies are not without risk or may be expensive and inconvenient to use.

Prescribing one of these preventive strategies, therefore, requires good reason for suspecting that the individual will develop osteoporosis. Some persons are more vulnerable than others. There are no laboratory tests that enable the medical community to predict with certainty who will and who won't develop the condition. Many of the factors that affect one's chances are known. Assessment of those factors can give an idea of overall risk. With this information, an individual and his or her physician can determine which approaches are best.

RISK FACTORS

Risk factors are the situations, characteristics, or conditions that can be associated with the likelihood of having a strong or a weak skeleton. For example, virtual absence of physical exercise, as when one is paralyzed, induces rapid loss of bone tissue. Hence, a prolonged period of bed rest enhances the likelihood of skeletal weakness. A condition that increases risk is not to be confused with a cause—scientists don't know how physical inactivity *causes* bone loss. If they did, physicians might be able to prevent that loss in bedridden individuals.

It is because bone mass, the amount of bone tissue, changes throughout life that risk factors come into play. Various factors influence how much bone tissue one accumulates during growth and during the continued strengthening and maturation of bones that occur even after one stops growing taller. Other factors influence the rate at which bone tissue is lost after the skeleton has fully matured.

Seven factors affect your chances of developing osteoporosis: age, genetics, hormones, calcium nutrition, lifestyle, medical illnesses and treatments, and drugs.

Age

The longer you live, the more likely you are to have osteoporosis. Osteoporosis afflicts more than one-half of individuals over the age of eighty, though there are sex and race differences (see below). Aging-associated osteoporosis reflects the relentless loss of skeletal tissue beginning well before the age of forty. The elderly are in double jeopardy for fracture. Their bones are weakened, and their chances of falling are increased, since balance reflexes are blunted with aging, balance-disrupting diseases are more common, and drugs that disturb balance are used more frequently. Hip fracture is the most common and the most devastating consequence of weak bones and falling, dramatically increasing in incidence between the ages of sixty-five and eighty-five. The risk of hip fracture extends to the elderly of both sexes, though not equally to each sex. Hip fractures are twice as likely to occur in women than in men.

Genetics

Sex, racial factors, and overall body size are determinants of bone mass and strength. Adult women have thinner, lighter bones than men at all ages and lose bone tissue more rapidly than men between the ages of fifty and sixty because of the reduced production of estrogen after menopause. The decrease in testosterone production in men as they age occurs more gradually and much later. Consequently, its effect on bone tissue is not apparent.

Race is a predictor of bone mass; Caucasians and Asians are more commonly afflicted with osteoporosis than blacks. Black people, in general, have heavier, thicker bones. Geographical residence in itself seems unrelated to risk for osteoporosis. For example, manifestations of osteoporosis are more common among European and American-born Jewish women residing in Jerusalem than among native-born Israeli women or women in the same site of African or Asian descent. South African blacks as well as American-born blacks have higher bone mass than their Caucasian counterparts. Body size, in part racially determined, also predicts the heaviness and strength of bone. Thin or petite individuals are more likely to manifest osteoporosis than their heavier counterparts. By contrast, large-framed, muscular, or obese people are less likely to have the condition.

Studies have indicated that fair-skinned, petite women of northern European extraction are at greatest risk for osteoporosis. Japanese women also appear to be at high risk, whereas osteoporosis is less common among women of Mediterranean origin. The predisposition of Asian peoples to osteoporosis may be due, at least partially, to their relatively small size. It must be stressed, however, that while there are population tendencies, there are so many individual exceptions that genetic prediction is far less than foolproof. Osteoporosis does occur in black women, and even in black men, though uncommonly.

There is evidence that having one or more blood relatives with osteoporosis increases one's chances of developing the condition. Perhaps this tendency is due to the inherited nature of other risk factors—such as race, body size, and the likelihood of surviving to a very old age.

Hormones

Estrogen and perhaps the other sex hormones (progesterone and testosterone) that direct sexual development and reproduction help prevent bone loss and protect against osteoporosis.

There is evidence that the extent of lifetime exposure to estrogen affects the amount of bone tissue, or bone mass, a woman will have in her later years. The longer and greater the exposure, the lower the risk of osteoporosis. Women are exposed to high levels of estrogen from puberty to menopause and to even higher levels during pregnancy. Use of oral contraceptives, which contain estrogens, increases exposure, as, of course, does estrogen use after menopause. Exposure of men to adult levels of testosterone starts at puberty and declines gradually after age seventy.

Women are at greater risk for osteoporosis than men, in part because they lose bone rapidly during the five- to ten-year period after menopause, the result of estrogen reduction. An average of 1–2 percent of bone tissue (even more in the spine) is lost each year in this accelerated phase. The longer a woman has lived after menopause, the greater her chances of having osteoporosis. The earlier the menopause, the earlier the acceleration of bone loss. Experiencing menopause well before the expected age, fifty-one years, could mean early osteoporosis. Premature menopause caused by surgical removal of both ovaries (bilateral oophorectomy), X-ray treatments for cancer, or ovarian diseases hasten the development of osteoporosis. Abrupt, complete loss of ovarian estrogen contrasts with the gradual and incomplete decreases of natural menopause, and swift, dramatic wasting of bone tissue results.

The age at onset of menstruation and also the number of full-term pregnancies help determine the duration of lifetime estrogen exposure, but their relationship to bone mass later on is unclear.

Some women are deprived of estrogen and progesterone temporarily during the childbearing years; excessive dieting (anorexia and bulimia) or a program of extremely vigorous physical training (as pursued by marathon runners and ballet dancers) may cause a "false

YOUR CHANCES OF DEVELOPING OSTEOPOROSIS

Increase as you get older

Are higher if you
- are a woman
- are white or Oriental
- had an early menopause
- are thin or petite
- have been paralyzed or bedridden
- have not had an adequate calcium intake
- have had part of your stomach or intestines removed
- smoke cigarettes
- drink alcohol in excess
- take a bone-wasting drug
- have an overactive thyroid gland

May be higher if you
- were deprived of female hormones before menopause or had no pregnancies
- have a blood relative with osteoporosis
- are intolerant of the milk sugar lactose

Are lower if you
- are obese or muscular
- have taken estrogen after menopause for more than one year

May be lower if you
- used oral contraceptives for more than one year
- had several pregnancies

---

menopause," in which the ovaries make too little estrogen and menstrual periods become irregular or stop. Bone loss ensues. The longer the situation continues, the greater the loss. Although some evidence indicates that bone tissue can be regained if menstruation returns to normal, it is not known whether recovery is complete. The menstrual cycle is a complex, precisely coordinated phenomenon that is easily disrupted by significant life stresses. Severe illness and even psychological stress can cause cessation of menstruation. Women who have had a long episode of false menopause when younger may have lost bone tissue. Another condition associated with estrogen and progesterone deficiency during childbearing years is prolactinoma. Prolactinoma is usually a noncancerous tumor of the pituitary gland that makes an excessive amount of the hormone prolactin. This hormone, normally involved in milk production during breast feeding after a pregnancy, also shuts off the ovaries. Women with prolactinoma have milk in their breasts without a prior pregnancy, stop menstruating, and lose bone tissue. Prolactinomas can be treated with drugs and surgery.

Men can also experience hormonal deficiency with the same skeletal consequences. Having one of the rare conditions in which there is a premature deficiency of testosterone or having a prolactinoma can provoke bone loss in younger men. Men with prolactinomas may notice discharge from their breasts; more commonly, however, their main symptom is impotence.

Calcium Nutrition

Adequate calcium nutrition is required to build strong bones during early life and help prevent excessive losses with advancing age. The body loses calcium when its intake is insufficient; calcium is not conserved. Consequently, calcium is withdrawn from its skeletal reservoir, and bone tissue is sacrificed.

Nevertheless, it is extremely difficult to prove scientifically that osteoporosis is a consequence of inadequate calcium nutrition. Everyone consumes some calcium, even if he or she avoids calcium-rich foods such as dairy products. Calcium needs vary from person to person and change at different times of life, and the differences between adequate and inadequate consumption may be small. Moreover, the effect of calcium deficiency is not as prominent or rapid as other factors that cause bone loss, such as postmenopausal estrogen reduction. Yet small differences, spread over many years, may make the difference between a healthy or an unhealthy skeleton at age sixty or seventy.

Some studies of large populations have shown that osteoporosis and osteoporosis-related fracture are more likely in people whose diets are low in calcium. In one such study, scientists examined the amount of bone tissue and the frequency of hip fracture in two separate Yugoslavian communities. In one community, people consumed an average of nearly 1,000 milligrams of calcium daily, chiefly by drinking milk. In the other, milk was not a regular part of the diet, and daily calcium consumption averaged about 500 milligrams. Those who consumed a large amount of calcium had heavier bones and fewer hip fractures than those who did not. Differences in calcium diet before the age of thirty were most important, supporting the idea that adequate calcium nutrition in the young is an investment in future bone health. Other studies have yielded similar results.

Lactose Intolerance
Individuals who have lactose intolerance, a condition that discourages milk drinking, seem more likely to develop osteoporosis. These people lack the digestive enzyme lactase—which breaks down the dairy sugar, lactose, in the intestines. Consequently, lactose-containing dairy products (milk, for example) cause disturbing symptoms such as bloating, gas, stomach cramps, and diarrhea, usually within fifteen to thirty minutes of consumption. It is the retention of undigested lactose in the intestines that is responsible for these symptoms. Because of their symptoms, people with lactase deficiency consume much less calcium in the form of dairy products than they should.

Lactose intolerance is particularly commonplace among the elderly, and as many as three-quarters of black, Asian, and Israeli adults have the condition, but no population is spared. For example, some studies have identified it in as many as one in five Caucasians of northern European ancestry. Lactose intolerance is also a feature of many types of intestinal disease.

The diagnosis of lactose intolerance, suspected because of the symptoms, is confirmed by simple laboratory tests. Patients can then be advised to eat certain dairy products that contain only small amounts of lactose or to take calcium supplements in pill or liquid form.

Lifestyle

Certain habits of everyday living such as physical exercise, use of alcohol, and cigarette smoking are also risk factors in the development of osteoporosis.

Insufficient Physical Exercise

Extreme physical immobility, as occurs in persons paralyzed from the neck down, induces rapid, severe loss of bone tissue from all parts of the skeleton. Individuals who are so immobilized can be expected to suffer 30 to 40 percent bone loss within several years. They commonly develop kidney stones, since the excess calcium released from bone is eliminated in the urine. Evidence indicates that bone is lost when there is insufficient antigravity exercise—exercise in which the limbs and body are moved against gravity's pull, such as walking and running. Immobilization of a limb in a plaster cast, for example, enhances loss of tissue from the bones of that limb. Exposure to zero gravity (weightlessness), as in space flight, produces a loss of bone tissue that resembles the losses caused by immobilization. Astronauts who were Skylab crew members lost an average of 2.5 percent of their bone tissue during their eighty-four days in space, amounting to a potential loss of 10 percent or more per year. It is not known whether a lack of exercise or some other effect of weightlessness caused the bone loss nor whether lost bone tissue is recovered upon return to normal gravity; some evidence indicates that recovery may not be complete.

Alcohol Abuse

Alcoholics are at high risk for fracture, partly because they are susceptible to falling and other injuries and partly because they have lost bone tissue. Skeletal weakening in alcoholics has many causes: liver disease, malnutrition, direct injury to bone-forming cells caused by alcohol, and alcohol's interference with calcium absorption. Also, alcoholism decreases estrogen production in women and testosterone production in men. The more alcohol habitually consumed, the greater the likelihood of osteoporosis. There is an increased risk of fracture among individuals who drink more than two ounces of hard liquor daily. Individuals who may not think they are alcoholics may be drinking enough to damage their bones.

Cigarette Smoking

Smoking has been implicated as a risk factor for many types of cancer, chronic bronchitis and emphysema, heart disease, and other illnesses. Smoking may also be a risk factor for osteoporosis and hip fracture. Some evidence indicates that smoking more than ten cigarettes per day for more than several years causes a loss of bone tissue; and smoking, together with other risk factors, such as being a thin or petite woman, appears to increase one's chances of breaking a hip in later life. Like the effects of alcohol on bone, those of smoking are not clear. Researchers do know that smoking interferes with the action of bone-protective hormones such as estrogen. There is evidence that women who smoke go through menopause an average of nearly two years earlier than nonsmokers. These are important reasons for you to stop smoking—and make sure your children and grandchildren get the message.

Medical Illnesses and Treatments

In as many as one in five women and one in three men who seek medical care because of existing osteoporosis—most often recognized by the presence of a fracture typical of the condition—some medical illness or treatment that may be a cause of the osteoporosis is also discovered; many respond to appropriate care. Consequently, their diagnosis is essential. Such conditions include hyperthyroidism, hyperparathyroidism, intestinal diseases and surgeries, rheumatoid arthritis, cancer, and osteomalacia. (See chapter 6 for a detailed discussion of these conditions.)

Drugs

Cortisone and several closely related hormones are manufactured by the adrenal glands, situated just above each kidney. These vital hormones are essential; they aid in preparing the body to meet severe stress, such as infection, and in storing a reserve supply of sugar. Scientists have known for nearly forty years that administration of high doses of these hormones or their more commonly used synthetic versions (corticosteroids) suppresses inflammation, helps prevent the rejection of transplanted organs, and blocks the growth of certain types of cancer. Consequently, they are indispensable drugs in treating a variety of medical disorders, including certain cancers, severe asthma, and some arthritic conditions.

Occasionally, the adrenal glands become overactive and release large amounts of cortisonelike chemicals into the bloodstream, a condition first described by Dr. Harvey Cushing and known as Cushing's syndrome.

Whether taken in high doses for medical purposes or made by overactive adrenals, these hormones produce many severe side effects, among them a dramatic loss of bone tissue. They poison bone-forming cells and stimulate the breakdown of bone tissue as well. Other side effects are diabetes mellitus, increased susceptibility to infection, wasting and weakness of muscles, mental disturbances, and a shift of body fat from the arms and legs to the trunk and face.

Osteoporosis can be expected to occur within five years of continuous exposure to high doses of cortisone or corticosteroids. Since exposure may be medically indicated and, indeed, lifesaving, physicians endeavor to minimize side effects by prescribing the lowest effective dose, every other day if possible, and gradually withdrawing the medication when it is no longer needed. Overactive adrenals can be treated effectively with surgery, irradiation, or drugs.

Evidence indicates that a high intake of calcium can help prevent osteoporosis in patients receiving corticosteroids; and other preventive approaches are now being tested, including the use of calcitonin and fluoride. Scientists are also testing a form of synthetic cortisone that is an effective treatment but does not damage the skeleton as much as other forms.

In addition to controlled use of corticosteroids, the use of thyroid pills, heparin (a blood thinner), and drugs that interfere with estrogen production should be monitored. Also, there are other drugs that appear to speed bone loss by diminishing the absorption of calcium from the diet or by promoting calcium excretion and are therefore risk factors in the development of osteoporosis. These include some antibiotics, laxatives, and water pills and are described in chapter 8.

PROTECTIVE FACTORS

Although the absence of risk factors—for example, being a man—may be regarded as protective, certain attributes or experiences sharply decrease the likelihood of developing osteoporosis and are considered protective factors. These include being obese or muscular and having experienced increased lifetime estrogen exposure.

Obesity

Obesity has been associated with a reduced incidence of osteoporosis. Although the degree of obesity needed for protection is unknown, one might expect that being 10 percent or more over ideal body weight is required. The reasons are not understood, but two possibilities are considered. First, significantly obese individuals have increased amounts of nonfat tissue—muscle and bone—perhaps because they must exert themselves more than thin people in pursuing the activities of daily living. Second, fatty tissue has the capacity to make estrogens, actually manufacturing them from the weak sex hormones of the adrenal glands. As a result, obese women are more likely than thin women to have bone-protective estrogen levels. Obesity has its own serious social drawbacks and medical complications (including diabetes mellitus, hypertension, heart disease, and an increased tendency to form dangerous blood clots) and does not guarantee the absence of osteoporosis—it only decreases the chances.

Muscularity

Being muscular may also protect. Muscularity implies a high level of exercise, which appears to benefit the skeleton. A muscular body build and heavy bones may be traits that are inherited together. There is also evidence that muscle, like fat, can synthesize estrogens—hardly an advantage for men but possibly protective in women. It should also be stressed that having good muscle tone may also help prevent injuries, such as falls, thereby decreasing the chances of breaking a bone. Thick muscle (or, for that matter, fat) may also afford a protective padding.

Estrogen Exposure

Increased premenopausal estrogen exposure has been suggested as but not proven to be a protective factor in women. Circumstances associated with increased estrogen exposure include a late menopause, completion of several pregnancies, and use of oral contraceptive pills for more than a year. These factors may be associated with an above-average bone mass at the time of menopause. Although a late menopause (mid-fifties or older) has not in itself been shown to protect, studies indicate that the number of years after menopause is an important determinant of bone mass in an individual. Hence, at any age, an older woman who had a late menopause is less likely to have osteoporosis than a woman who experienced an early menopause (mid-forties or younger); the difference is most likely due to the number of years a woman is devoid of the protective effect of premenopausal estrogen levels. Whether pregnancy and oral contraceptive use are protective is controversial; clear advantages remain to be established. Even if women who have had several pregnancies and/or used birth control pills do accumulate more bone tissue before menopause, as has been suggested, estrogen may not be responsible. Certainly, pregnancy is accompanied by high estrogen levels, and oral contraceptive pills contain estrogens. Yet other factors may explain possible differences in the bone mass of menopausal women—variations in lifestyle, for example (general nutrition, exercise, smoking, and alcohol intake).

Pregnancy

The suspicion that pregnancy is protective may come as a surprise to some readers, since the mother's skeleton is commonly regarded as a source of calcium to build the fetus's bones. Although a pregnant woman does need more calcium, hormonal changes increase the ability of the intestine to absorb calcium from the diet; the calcium a pregnant woman consumes, therefore, is used more efficiently. As a result, skeletal calcium stores tend to be preserved, provided calcium intake is adequate. At the same time, the large amounts of estrogen and other hormones made by the placenta may act to reduce bone loss.

Estrogen Therapy

Finally, postmenopausal estrogen use has been proven to reduce bone loss. This fact is the basis for treating women with estrogens to prevent osteoporosis. (See chapter 11 for a detailed discussion of estrogen therapy.)

6 • Medical Causes of Osteoporosis

A number of medical conditions increase the risk of developing osteoporosis and must be carefully supervised by a physician so that bone loss is prevented or minimized.

HYPERTHYROIDISM

Exposure to too much thyroid hormone (hyperthyroidism) accelerates bone loss and can, after several years, cause osteoporosis. The thyroid hormones—thyroxine, or T_4, and triiodothyronine, or T_3—control the metabolic rate. This refers to how rapidly foods are burned, or metabolized, and thereby are converted to energy for all bodily functions and for the maintenance of a normal body temperature.

One can be exposed to an excessive amount of thyroid hormone in two ways: having an overactive thyroid gland and taking too much thyroid hormone in pill form. Thyroid gland overactivity can arise from a disturbance in the regulation of hormone output or from inflammation or tumor within the gland itself. The most common regulatory disruption in the young is called Graves' disease, in which the thyroid gland becomes overactive and may be enlarged. Individuals with Graves' disease may also have bulging eyes and problems with vision. In older people, noncancerous thyroid tumors are the most common cause of hyperthyroidism.

The only justification for taking thyroid pills is to compensate for a failing or underactive thyroid gland (hypothyroidism) or to shrink or prevent the growth of certain kinds of abnormal thyroid tissue. Unfortunately, taking too much thyroid medication is a form of drug abuse. Thyroid hormone is a stimulant and is sometimes prescribed to promote weight loss. This is an ill-conceived, dangerous undertaking that promotes the loss of muscle and bone tissue as well as fat and can be fatal. Adjusting the dose of thyroid hormone in hypothyroidism is difficult; some patients are inadvertently overtreated.

Hyperthyroidism, regardless of cause, can produce symptoms such as discomfort in warm environments, nervousness, sweating, weight loss despite an increased appetite, weakness, tiredness, and palpitations (pounding, racing heartbeat) or skipped heartbeats. Some hyperthyroid individuals, particularly the elderly, experience only muscle weakness or palpitations, or, alternatively, depression or apathy—a condition known as apathetic or "masked" hyperthyroidism.

The more severe or prolonged the hyperthyroidism, the more likely is significant bone loss. Osteoporosis is a particular danger among postmenopausal women or the elderly who are hyperthyroid; the combination of factors sharply increases risk.

Hyperthyroidism must be recognized and treated—not only to protect the skeleton but also to prevent other complications, such as heart disease and severe muscle weakness. Typical symptoms and physical findings point the physician to the diagnosis; confirmation comes from the results of laboratory tests. Thyroid pills should be withdrawn from abusers. Radioactive iodine therapy, surgery, and antithyroid medications are used to control an overactive thyroid gland.

HYPERPARATHYROIDISM

Parathyroid hormone prevents the level of calcium in the blood from falling too low. Its release repairs blood calcium deficiency by promoting calcium removal from bone tissue and absorption from the diet. Restoration of a normal blood calcium level shuts off parathyroid hormone production.

One or more parathyroid glands may enlarge and become overactive, immune to the normal shutoff mechanism. This condition, known as hyperparathyroidism, causes a dangerous, persistent rise in blood calcium. Wasting of bone tissue, stomach pain, kidney stones, and mental dysfunction can result.

Hyperparathyroidism is not rare. Mild forms are unexpectedly discovered through routine laboratory examination in one of every 1,000 patients admitted to a hospital. Since hyperparathyroidism may not cause symptoms, bone loss may produce unsuspected osteoporosis. Most common in middle-aged women, hyperparathyroidism can combine with the menopause to increase the risk of osteoporosis markedly.

Treatment of hyperparathyroidism with surgery to remove the enlarged glands is almost always successful.

INTESTINAL DISEASES AND SURGERIES

The digestive, or gastrointestinal, tract is an engineering marvel that reduces foodstuffs into their component nutrients, dissolves them, and transports them into the body. Digestion actually begins in the mouth; chewing mixes food with saliva, which contains some digestive enzymes. The food particles travel via the esophagus into the stomach, where digestion begins in earnest through the action of stomach acid and more digestive enzymes. Absorption of some nutrients occurs in the stomach, but most absorption takes place in the lengthy small intestine—aided by the further digestive action of enzymes from the pancreas and by bile, which prepares fats for absorption. Finally, the colon, or large intestine, removes water from the digestive residue, leaving waste products that are excreted as stool.

Malabsorption is the medical condition in which the absorptive function of the gastrointestinal tract is not properly carried out. It has many causes including surgical removal of part of the stomach or intestine; abuse of laxatives; intestinal infection; intestinal tumors; a condition known as sprue, in which exposure to the wheat protein gluten (also found in rye, barley, and oats) damages the intestine; and disorders of the pancreas. People who have malabsorption may have no symptoms at all, in which case their problem goes unrecognized. More commonly, however, malabsorption symptoms include diarrhea; consistent passing of large amounts of greasy, foul-smelling, silver-colored (because it contains undigested fats) stool; weight loss; anemia; muscle and joint pains; and a tendency to bleed too easily and too long at sites of injury.

From the standpoint of bone health, gastrointestinal diseases can interfere with the absorption of calcium and vitamin D. Having part of the stomach removed to decrease acid production when ulcers are present can reduce the absorption of calcium, leading to bone loss. Malabsorption of calcium and vitamin D in patients with severe intestinal or pancreatic diseases can produce osteoporosis. If severe and prolonged, osteomalacia may be the result. This condition of soft bones results from a drastic deficiency of calcium and phosphorus; there is not enough mineral to calcify and therefore harden the bones. The active form of vitamin D may have a direct hardening effect on bones as well. In childhood, osteomalacia is called rickets, and the soft bones of children with rickets are often immature and deformed.

It is important to recognize malabsorption, since many of its causes can be treated with proper diet; oral administration of enzyme pills, calcium, and vitamin D; and other methods. Individuals with gastrointestinal disorders can avoid bone disease.

RHEUMATOID ARTHRITIS

Rheumatoid arthritis (RA) is a chronic inflammation of the joints that may lead to deformity and loss of joint function. It is more common in women than in men and occurs mainly after the age of thirty. Typically, patients with RA experience many episodes of swelling, pain, redness, and stiffness in the joints of the hands, feet, wrists, and knees, though virtually any joint can be involved. Skin rash, anemia, numbness, muscle weakness, and other complications may occur as well. Physical therapy and anti-inflammatory drugs are first lines of treatment, though other agents are used in more severe, long-lasting cases. Occasionally, patients are treated with corticosteroids. Bone loss may occur in these patients because of the prolonged inflammation and the immobility that the disease causes and as a complication of treatment with these drugs. For these reasons, it is crucial that afflicted patients be treated effectively and that corticosteroids be used as infrequently as possible. Maintaining mobility and adequate calcium nutrition are extremely important.

CANCER

Certain types of cancer arise in bone marrow cells, contained within bone, and erode adjacent bone tissue. The most common of these, representing about 1 percent of all cancers, is multiple myeloma, in which a particular strain of marrow cell, the plasma cell, becomes cancerous and destroys bone. Cancerous plasma cells are known to produce a chemical called OAF, or Osteoclast Activating Factor, a powerful stimulator of bone-dissolving osteoclasts. Multiple myeloma occurs principally in middle age or later—the average age is sixty. Patients with multiple myeloma often have severe osteoporosis; in fact, a fracture may be the first symptom of the disease, though anemia and frequent infections, such as pneumonia, may also announce its presence. Although incurable, multiple myeloma is treatable; special anticancer drugs can prolong life and prevent symptoms. Other types of cancers that erode the skeleton include mastocytosis—a rare proliferation of cells that inhabit the bone marrow, the skin, and other organs. These cancer cells produce heparin, a naturally occurring anticoagulant that causes bone loss. Doctors use heparin as a blood thinner in certain medical conditions; when its use is prolonged, bone loss can result. Cancers that reach bone from other organs, such as the lungs, by the bloodstream (metastases) may also cause osteoporosis.

OTHER DISEASES

Osteoporosis has been reported to occur along with other medical disorders, including chronic obstructive pulmonary disease, commonly known as emphysema, and certain kinds of liver and kidney diseases. Heavy cigarette smoking, a causative factor in emphysema, may be the reason for bone loss in that condition. Decreased absorption of calcium by the intestine may explain the loss of bone tissue in some patients with severe liver disease. Diabetes mellitus has been suggested as a risk factor for osteoporosis, but this is still being debated. Acromegaly, a rare disease originating with a pituitary tumor in which facial features become coarse and the hands and feet enlarge, leads to osteoporosis. Finally, several hereditary disorders are associated with thin bones and fractures—osteoporosis that usually appears in childhood. The most common of these hereditary diseases is osteogenesis imperfecta, or brittle bone disease. A national society, the Brittle Bone Society, sponsors vital communication among patients and families of patients and raises money needed for patient care and research.

OSTEOMALACIA—A CONDITION THAT MIMICS OSTEOPOROSIS

Osteomalacia is characterized by a softening of bone tissue. It usually arises because of a severe deficiency of vitamin D or a failure of vitamin D to act in the body. As a result, not enough calcium and phosphorus are provided to harden bones. Vitamin D may also have an effect on the hardening process, quite apart from its role as a mineral provider. Mild vitamin D deficiency appears to produce a calcium deficit that does not soften bones but speeds up bone loss and can increase the risk of osteoporosis.

This serious problem leads to very small fractures that do not heal well and cannot be seen on ordinary X-ray pictures. Other symptoms of osteomalacia are severe weakness—particularly difficulty in climbing stairs, standing up from a bed or chair, or sitting up in bed—and pains that doctors often confuse with arthritis, sciatica, or rheumatic backaches. The diagnosis of osteomalacia is made by blood tests and by analyzing samples of bone tissue (bone biopsy).

Osteomalacia has many causes: not eating an adequate amount of vitamin D and avoiding sunlight; disorders of the liver or kidneys that impair the processing of vitamin D so that it fails to act in the body; and intestinal diseases characterized by malabsorption of vitamin D, calcium, and phosphorus. Why mention osteomalacia? First, osteomalacia may look the same as osteoporosis on X rays of the bones, yet its treatment is entirely different. Second, there is reason to believe that osteomalacia is not uncommon among housebound elderly who are not eating well and are not exposed to much sunlight. Third, the soft bones of osteomalacia and the brittle bones of osteoporosis, combined in some older people, may heighten the risk of fracture. Remember, a mild state of vitamin D deficiency itself may cause osteoporosis. Fourth, when deficiency of vitamin D is the cause of osteomalacia, vitamin D administration is the cure.

7 • Measuring Bone Mass

Just by feeling, one can estimate the size of some parts of the skeleton, such as the bones of the forearm and shin. But the size of these bones has little to do with their strength; larger or longer bones are not necessarily stronger. Two factors are more important: the amount of bone tissue inside the bone itself (bone mass or calcium content) and the quality of that bone tissue. Two bones of the same size may differ markedly in strength. The weaker bone will contain a thinner cortical shell and less spongy bone. It will be hollower and therefore have a lower bone mass. Moreover, the bony tissue it contains may be abnormal and unhealthy. In osteoporosis, internal tissue is usually lost from all bones, including the bones of the arms and legs, the ribs, the skull, the mandible (jaw bone), vertebrae (the spine), and the pelvis. In some instances, normal tissue may be replaced by unhealthy tissue.

If one can't appreciate the mass and strength of a bone just by inspecting its outer dimensions, how can a physician determine whether an individual might be at risk for or already have osteoporosis? How can the response to treatment be detected? How can scientists study the causes of osteoporosis and discover new ways to prevent and treat it? Remember, the loss of bone tissue leading to osteoporosis is gradual and silent—and osteoporosis itself has no symptoms unless there is a fracture. Also recognize that there is presently no blood or urine test that can help physicians detect osteoporosis, though tests are being developed that may allow doctors to determine how fast bone is disappearing. Many mistakenly assume that X rays are the answer—a logical idea, since X rays detect broken bones and probe the internal structures of the body. Although ordinary X rays used for diagnostic purposes can reveal fractures typical of osteoporosis, such as a crushed vertebra or a broken wrist or hip, they are not very helpful in determining bone mass. By the time fractures occur, much bone tissue has already been lost. More sophisticated X-ray methods are necessary.

What techniques are available to assist the physician in detecting bone loss *before* a fracture is likely to occur? How do physicians determine whether treatment is working? Several methods are now available. In selecting the best method, a physician must evaluate each method with respect to its *precision, accuracy,* and *sensitivity.*

Precision refers to the ability of a method to give the same results in the same individual when it is repeated in several days to weeks; high precision means that the results are consistent. Doctors don't test people frequently over a short period of time; they occasionally use short-term measurements to make sure that the method works. A high degree of precision allows physicians to detect the small changes in bone mass that may occur over a period of six months to one year.

An *accurate* bone measurement determines the amount of bone tissue, or amount of calcium, in the bone measured. One would get the same result if the bone were removed from the body and analyzed for calcium.

A *sensitive* procedure easily distinguishes people with early osteoporosis from those who are of identical age and sex but do not have osteoporosis.

In considering X-ray methods for measuring bone mass, physicians, scientists, *and* patients are concerned with radiation exposure. Extremely high doses of radiation, as might occur following a nuclear attack or an accident in a nuclear energy plant, cause sickness and death or, if the dose is less extreme but still high, cancer, sterilization, or genetic abnormalities. The tissue-damaging properties of X rays have been harnessed for use in treating certain medical conditions, such as cancer. Similarly beneficial are modern X-ray methods used for diagnosis, which provide *very low* radiation exposure—a large number of routine X-ray studies would still not be expected to harm an individual. Yet the effects of radiation on the body are cumulative—they add up and never diminish or disappear—and unnecessary exposure must be avoided.

A routine X ray, as might be used to examine the chest or detect a broken bone, is not precise, accurate, or sensitive enough to detect early osteoporosis in very susceptible bone, such as the spine. An individual will have to lose as much as 40 percent of the bone mass (calcium) before it becomes obvious on a routine X ray of the spine! Moreover, an individual receives ten to fifteen times the radiation exposure from a spinal X ray than from an ordinary chest X ray. The reasons for the poor diagnostic value of standard X rays are many: the X-ray technician may fail to position the person properly; an individual may be exposed to the X ray for different periods of time during the test, and different types of X-ray photographic film may be used, which produce varying results when the X ray is developed. Think about how difficult it is for different individuals to obtain the same photographs with different cameras, different film, and different film-processing procedures. However, if a vertebra has become partially fractured, as is easily seen on a spinal X ray, subsequent X rays can be used to see how fast the vertebra shrinks to the point where it is crushed completely simply by measuring with a ruler the change in the height of the fractured vertebra.

Recently, modified X-ray procedures have become available that offer much better precision, accuracy, and sensitivity than the routine X ray and expose the patient to very low levels of radiation. These methods were designed to measure bone in the arms and legs and in the spine and are called Single Photon Absorptiometry (SPA), Dual Photon Absorptiometry (DPA), and Computed Axial Tomography (CAT).

SINGLE PHOTON ABSORPTIOMETRY (SPA)

The procedure for the SPA measurement is quite simple and takes no more than twenty to twenty-five minutes. The arm that is not used to write or eat is placed in a water bath or wrapped in a blood-pressure-like cuff; a small unit containing a radioactive material scans the arm, usually at the wrist end. Similar SPA units are used to measure the amount of bone in the heel. The amount of bone in the area scanned immediately appears on a computer printout. Since the radiation exposure SPA provides is so minute (one-fifth the radiation of a chest X ray) and because its precision is high, SPA can be used repeatedly. It is often used at intervals as short as three to four months to follow the responses of patients to treatment and to determine how fast bone tissue is disappearing in high-risk individuals, such as those receiving a synthetic cortisonelike drug (see chapter 5). On average, SPA costs $60 to $95 per measurement. Unfortunately, there are two problems with SPA.

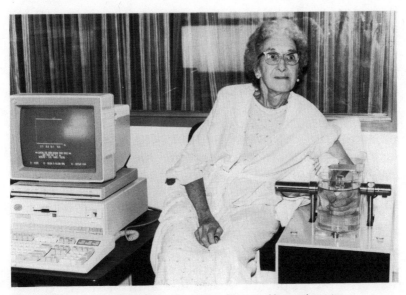

Measurement of Bone Mass with Single Photon Absorptiometry

First, measurements of the forearm or heel bones cannot be used to predict who is at risk for spinal bone loss, which ultimately causes the most common osteoporosis-related fractures in postmenopausal women. This is primarily because the forearm bones contain a large amount of cortical tissue that is not lost as fast as the spongy bone of the vertebrae. Losses of bone from the vertebrae cannot be detected by measurements of the forearm. The limits of this technique should be stressed, since a number of so-called diagnostic clinics recommend SPA measurements alone as a means to detect individuals at risk for vertebral fractures. A second problem also must be recognized. It is not certain whether SPA results apply to the hip, another place commonly devastated by osteoporosis. However, even though SPA of forearm or heel does not disclose the bone mass of the spine and hip, these different bones generally respond the same way to treatment, so SPA can be used to tell whether treatment is working.

DUAL PHOTON ABSORPTIOMETRY (DPA)

By contrast with SPA, dual photon absorptiometry (DPA) measures the bone mass of the spine and hip, the bones in which mass is most critical medically. The cost of measurement is high, typically ranging from $130 to $200. Previously available only in large hospitals, DPA equipment is becoming more widespread and is being used in outpatient departments and clinics. Like SPA, DPA is easy to perform and causes no patient discomfort. It takes about thirty to forty minutes. A device scans the bones, such as the vertebrae; records the amount of tissue; and prints out the data for evaluation. The radiation dose one receives from DPA is also small (one-fifth the radiation of a routine chest X ray and much less than that from the very insensitive routine spinal X-ray procedure). DPA measures *all* the calcium in its path. Unfortunately, this means that in spinal studies, the results can be erroneous; some older patients have extra calcium deposits around the vertebrae, as part of wear-and-tear arthritis, as well as calcium deposits in blood vessels due to hardening of the arteries, or arteriosclerosis.

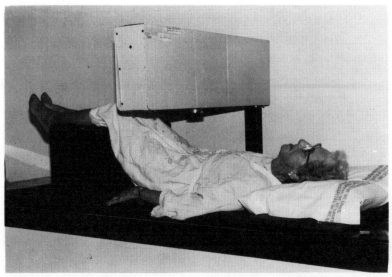
Bone Mass Being Measured with Dual Photon Absorptiometry

COMPUTED AXIAL TOMOGRAPHY (CAT)

Although CAT measurement of bone mass in the vertebrae is relatively new, CAT-scanning procedures have been used routinely for many years to study the spine for the presence of slipped discs and bone tumors. This new CAT technique actually measures the bone tissue in the center of each vertebra; it is the spongy bone in this area that is most susceptible to osteoporosis. Extra calcium around the spine, due to arthritis or arteriosclerosis, does not affect the results. Although a CAT study gives approximately fifty times more radiation than a DPA study, that is still one-third less than the dose received from a routine X ray of the spine, which, as noted earlier, has *limited diagnostic value* for detecting osteoporosis before the vertebrae fracture. The cost for CAT measurement of vertebral bone mass ranges from $200 to $300.

When used to study large groups of people, both CAT and DPA demonstrate the gradual loss of spinal bone, which begins at thirty to thirty-five years of age in women

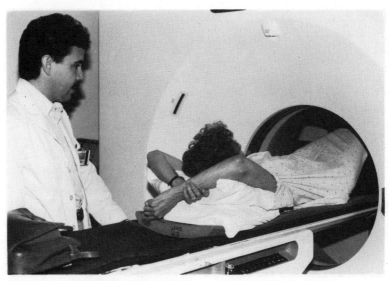
Measurement of Bone Mass with Computed Axial Tomography

and proceeds at approximately 0.5 to 1 percent per year. Losses accelerate to 2 to 3 percent per year during the five to ten years that follow the menopause. CAT and DPA procedures have shown that men lose approximately 20–30 percent of their spinal bone during their lifetime after age thirty (more than half of which occurs after age sixty). On the other hand, women lose 45—50 percent of the bone tissue from their vertebrae during their lifetime, the greater percentage between age forty-five and sixty.

Although good for studying groups of people, currently available DPA and CAT procedures are still not sensitive enough to detect the *risk* of osteoporosis developing *in any one individual,* nor are they reliable enough to detect small changes in an individual's bones. They are not sensitive enough for screening people with little or no deficiency in bone mass to determine their chances of developing osteoporosis and cannot be used to determine how fast one is losing bone tissue unless the losses are considerable. Usually, intervals of two to three years between tests are needed to diagnose the speed of bone loss.

On the other hand, either DPA or CAT can be used to diagnose existing osteoporosis (or a low bone mass). A woman whose bone mass is on the low side at menopause is at great risk for severe osteoporosis later on. A new DPA technique, called Dual Energy Radiography or Quantitative Digital Radiography, has been developed that gives promise of greater reliability—and lower cost.

Beware of those who advertise routine and simple evaluation of bone mass with SPA as a predictive test for spinal fractures. It is a waste of money! Analyze your risk factors and seek the opinion of qualified members of the medical profession who will then determine if a measurement of vertebral bone mass is required, with either DPA or CAT procedures, and honestly analyze the cost-effectiveness of the procedure for you.

NEUTRON ACTIVATION

Neutron activation, which measures the total amount of calcium in the body, is an even more complex X-ray method. Since almost all calcium is in bone, the measurement indicates the amount of bone calcium. Highly sophisticated, expensive equipment is needed; the test is available at few health centers and is used mainly for research.

BIOPSY

Another way to diagnose osteoporosis is to take a biopsy sample of bone tissue and study it under the microscope. Biopsy of bone does not require surgery but rather is performed by inserting under local anesthesia a wide-bore hollow needle and obtaining a core of bone tissue, usually from the pelvis. Biopsied tissue can indicate whether osteoporosis is present, and, if so, whether there is a cause for the osteoporosis, such as cancer of the bone marrow; it can also indicate whether the patient has osteomalacia (see chapter 6). Most patients do not need a bone biopsy for diagnosis—generally evaluation of medical history, family history, and current state of health and measurement of bone mass are enough. Bone biopsy is done only when secondary osteoporosis or osteomalacia is suspected and cannot be proved by medical examination. Expertise is required to do the biopsy and process the sample appropriately. Although bone biopsy does reflect the amount of bone tissue at the biopsy site, it does not indicate the mass of bone in other parts of the skeleton.

MEASURING BONE MASS

Method	Area Studied
Single Photon Absorptiometry (SPA)	Forearm, Heel
Dual Photon Absorptiometry (DPA)	Spine, Hip, Other Bones, and the Amount of Calcium in the Entire Body
Computed Axial Tomography (CAT)	Spine

8 • Strengthening Bone Through Diet

Calcium is essential for the entire body, not just the bones, to function properly. It must be included as a dietary nutrient, since the body cannot manufacture it. Although the skeleton stores calcium, those stores shrink and the bones weaken when calcium intake is insufficient or the absorption of calcium is compromised. Just consuming an adequate amount of calcium is not enough to maintain strong bones; general nutritional habits must be good, and there must be enough vitamin D either by sunlight exposure or in the diet to allow the intestine to absorb the calcium ingested.

NORMAL CALCIUM CONSUMPTION

The United States government recommends that nonpregnant adults consume an average of 800 milligrams of calcium daily (the amount of calcium in two and two-thirds eight-ounce glasses of milk). This is the so-called Recommended Dietary Allowance (RDA) developed by the U.S. Committee on Dietary Allowances of the Food and Nutrition Board. Higher levels are recommended for adolescents and for pregnant women (1,200 milligrams daily, the equivalent of four eight-ounce glasses of milk).

There are RDA standards for many nutrients including vitamins and minerals. Based on available scientific knowledge, they indicate what is good nutrition for almost all healthy people. The RDAs are not individual requirements, since medical conditions and the use of drugs may affect a person's needs. Rather, they are recommendations for the daily amounts of nutrients that specific populations should consume over a period of time to satisfy the requirements of 97 percent of those groups (see the RDA established for minerals on page 78). They should only be used as general guidelines; people with medical conditions should consult their physician and dietitian to assess their own special requirements.

There is another set of dietary standards. The United States Recommended Daily Allowance (USRDA) was established by the Food and Drug Administration (FDA) to be used in the nutritional labeling of the general food supply and for labeling special dietary foods and dietary supplements. Unlike the RDA, which makes separate recommendations for seventeen different groups of people (different ages and sexes), the USRDA acknowledges only four population groups, according to age (see page 76). The USRDA for calcium is 1,000 milligrams daily. The recommendations used on most nutrition labels are for children over four years of age and adults.

Many nutritionists suspect that the calcium RDA of 800 milligrams is too low. This is because the RDA was based primarily on studies in younger people, whereas older people have difficulty in utilizing dietary calcium. Normally, the body can adjust to a low-calcium diet; it actually increases the proportion of dietary calcium it absorbs. This adjustment, called adaptation, diminishes with increasing age. In other words, a young, fully grown person needs less calcium than an older person; an older person needs to eat more calcium to guarantee a bone-protective intake. Although adaptation is not completely understood, researchers recognize changes with aging that could explain the higher calcium needs of the older adult.

AMOUNT OF CALCIUM NEEDED

There are strong indications that many adults need 1,000 milligrams daily (the USRDA for calcium) on the average and, as they enter their fifties, sixties, and beyond, as much as 1,500 milligrams per day, or the calcium in six glasses of milk, if they are at high risk for osteoporosis. Studies have indicated that one can actually lose more calcium from the body than one gains (negative calcium balance) when diets contain less than 1,000 milligrams a day (see chapter 4). Negative balance for a long period of time (more than a few months) can cause *loss of bone tissue,* since most of the calcium in the body is stored in bone! *As emphasized at a 1987 conference cosponsored by the National Institutes of Health and the National Osteoporosis Foundation, the amount of calcium needed to prevent negative balance varies among different individuals. One should consume 1,000 milligrams daily to minimize the potential of developing a negative calcium balance. People at high risk for osteoporosis may need as much as 1,500 milligrams daily.*

Dietary surveys (HANES—Health and Nutrition Examination Survey, I and II) performed by the United States Department of Health, Education and Welfare indicate that most people consume less than the RDA for calcium, and many far less, even though the RDA is probably too low. This observation is well supported by several findings:

- More than two-thirds of women between adolescence and age thirty-five consume less calcium than the RDA, just as the skeleton is maturing and requires calcium to become as strong as possible. Those women who fail to make all the bone they can may gradually develop osteoporosis later on (make sure your children and grandchildren know this).
- After age thirty-five, three-quarters of all women consume less than the RDA during any given day. In fact, many have a daily intake of less than 300 milligrams.
- Older people, who need more calcium, are most likely to be consuming less than the recommended amount of calcium.
- The diets of one-third of adults are deficient in calcium.
- Calcium deficiency in adults is much more common than iron deficiency.

REASONS FOR INADEQUATE CALCIUM INTAKE

Calcium deficiency may be just one part of an overall nutritional problem in individuals as they age.

Change in Food Habits

Food habits may deteriorate with aging, for many reasons:

- One may avoid milk. Many older adults have long since lost the habit of drinking milk, despite the fact that milk (and other dairy products) is the main source of dietary calcium. Some do not like its taste or want its calories and fat (even though skim milk contains slightly more calcium than whole milk); some can't tolerate it, either because of lactose intolerance (see chapter 5) or, rarely, a definite allergy to milk. Allergy to milk—with skin rashes, wheezing, and other problems—is much more common in children than in adults.

- Fewer calories are needed to meet energy needs (see page 63). Energy needs of adult females decrease from 2,000 calories per day at twenty-three to fifty years of age to 1,800 calories per day at fifty-one to seventy-five years of age. After age seventy-five, the energy needs drop to 1,600 calories per day. As one eats less, one's intake of certain vital nutrients may also decrease, even though needs have not changed or have actually increased.

- Economic problems influence eating habits. Currently, one-fifth of people sixty-five years of age or older are poor. Food with high nutritional value can be expensive.

- Physical and social isolation is also a problem. Lonely people can become depressed and lose the desire to eat properly. According to a recent survey conducted for the Commonwealth Fund Commission on people sixty-five and older living in households, 39 percent of women and 16 percent of men were living alone (a total of 8.3 million of the estimated 27.6 million people in this category).

- Decreased enjoyment of food can also cause poor nutrition. Some loss of taste and smell that accompanies aging makes eating less satisfying. Loss of taste can also prompt certain poor eating habits, such as the use of large amounts of salt and sugar to make food more tasty.
- Poor teeth and gums and loss of teeth prevent thorough chewing and thus limit a wide selection of foods. Approximately 25 million Americans are completely without teeth, and tooth loss increases with advancing age. Dentures don't help necessarily, since they can further diminish taste and may not fit well enough to allow normal chewing.

  Smokers are much more likely than nonsmokers to need dentures after the age of fifty. Fewer nonsmokers without osteoporosis than those with osteoporosis have required dentures. Middle-aged women may be more likely to keep their teeth if they avoid smoking and follow nutritional habits that are designed to prevent the progression of osteoporosis.
- Chronic diseases—such as arthritis, heart failure, and diabetes—and certain drugs can depress the appetite

ENERGY AND PROTEIN NEEDS OF ADULTS

	Age	Energy (calories)	Protein (grams)
Men	19–22	2,900	56
	23–50	2,700	56
	51–75	2,400	56
	over 75	2,050	56
Women	15–22	2,100	46
	23–50	2,000	44
	51–75	1,800	44
	over 75	1,600	44

Adapted from *Recommended Dietary Allowances*, 9th ed., Washington, D.C., National Academy of Sciences, 1980.

or require individuals to follow special diets that make eating undesirable. Laxatives and diuretics (drugs that stimulate the kidneys to eliminate salt and water) contribute to the problem, as do low-salt diets.

- Alcohol provides empty, nonnutritional calories, thus suppressing appetite and causing deficiency of essential vitamins and minerals. When used in excess, it can impair the absorption of calcium from the intestine.

Increase in Calcium Needs

Drugs and dietary habits may further increase calcium needs. Among such drugs are thyroid hormone preparations and corticosteroids taken in excess; certain drugs used to treat epilepsy; certain antacid preparations containing aluminum that are commonly taken for ulcers or heartburn and increase the loss of calcium in the urine; some antibiotics, such as tetracycline taken regularly, especially just before or after a meal; and certain diuretics that cause the loss of calcium from your body.

Older people need more calcium than younger people for many reasons. They cannot adjust to a diet that is low in calcium. Most of these reasons relate to vitamin D, the vitamin that is needed for absorption of calcium from the foods you eat.

Individuals over age sixty-five—

- may get less sunlight, particularly if they live in a cold climate or spend much of their time indoors for other reasons; therefore, the skin will make less vitamin D.
- may become vitamin D–deficient even if sunlight exposure occurs, since elderly people do not produce the same amount of vitamin D in the skin as younger people exposed to the same amount of sunlight.
- do not convert vitamin D to its active form in the kidney as thoroughly as younger people.
- may not get enough vitamin D in their diet.
- are more likely to be using drugs that interfere with calcium absorption and cause calcium wasting: some

drugs used to treat epilepsy, thyroid hormone or corticosteroids in excess, aluminum-containing antacids (often used for heartburn), and certain antibiotics, such as tetracycline.
- have experienced loss, if they are women, of estrogens due to menopause, which decreases the ability to adjust to a calcium-poor diet.

Lack of vitamin D can injure the skeleton in two ways: (1) the calcium deficiency that results can produce *osteoporosis*, as calcium is released from its bony storehouse to satisfy the body's needs; and (2) calcium deficiency plus *severe* vitamin D deficiency causes *osteomalacia* (see chapter 6).

Decrease in Calcium Gains

Dietary factors may decrease calcium gains. Diets high in fat, fiber, or bran or that contain certain chemical agents (phytates) can bind calcium in the intestine and prevent its absorption into the body. For example, an increase in fiber intake of 26 grams increases calcium requirement by 150 milligrams per day. Diets that contain excessive amounts of protein, carbohydrate, caffeinated coffee or other beverages, and salt may also increase your calcium requirements by causing a calcium drain in the urine. A habit of more than two or three cups of caffeinated coffee daily can cause significant calcium wasting over time. Strict vegetarians, especially those who avoid milk and eggs, may be eating too much fiber and may not be getting enough vitamin D and therefore not absorbing calcium properly.

CALCIUM CONTENT OF FOODS

An average United States diet consists primarily of four essential food groups:

- A milk-dairy group, which supplies 70–75 percent of the calcium available for eating. If one excludes dairy products from the diet, the calcium intake averages only 300 milligrams per day.

- A meat and fish group, which is the source of 10 percent of the dietary calcium.
- A fruit-vegetable group, which offers only 10 percent of the calcium to the diet.
- A bread, nut, and grain group, which supplies less than 5 percent of the calcium.

Fresh milk, powdered milk, buttermilk, cottage cheese, and milk puddings should be avoided if you have lactase deficiency, since they all contain a considerable amount of lactose. Remember, too, that a variety of other foods contain dairy products. If the word *parve* or *pareve* is on the package, you can assume that the food does not contain any dairy product (the word *pareve* refers to neutral foods—such as fish, eggs, fruits, and vegetables—that are permissible to use with meat or milk meals according to orthodox Jewish dietary laws). Low-fat yogurt, which contains 300 milligrams of calcium per cup, can also be tolerated by some individuals with lactose intolerance. Not only is yogurt low in lactose, but it also contains lactase (deficient in people with lactose intolerance), which helps digest the lactose. This enzyme exists only in yogurt that has not been pasteurized. Keep sodium in mind when you decide to drink buttermilk or eat yogurt. Both of these foods have more sodium per eight-ounce serving than milk.

Eating fermented milk products (yogurt, for example) or drinking regular milk in small quantities during the day often makes it easier to use milk as a source of calcium if you have lactase deficiency. Remember, one absorbs more calcium from a pint of milk if the milk is taken in five to six portions during the day than if all the milk in the pint is taken at one stitting. Lactose-free ice cream, milks, and cheeses are also available. However, these products are expensive and also have a much sweeter taste than regular cow's milk. Tolerance to lactose can be increased by adding the enzyme lactase in either tablet or liquid forms to milk eighteen to twenty-four hours before drinking it.

In general, the calcium content of meat is quite low—though alligator meat is an excellent source, containing 1,200 milligrams of calcium per serving. A meat-rich diet may actually prove harmful to calcium reserves in the skeleton, since excessive meat protein intake can increase calcium losses in the urine. For instance, Eskimos, whose diet is extremely high in meat, have less bone than non-Eskimos. Certain fish, such as sardines and salmon, are rich in calcium, but to benefit from the high calcium content, you must also eat the bones!

Increasingly, manufacturers are adding calcium to foods such as cereals, flour, and colas. Several fruit drinks are now on the market that are enriched with calcium that is known to be particularly well absorbed from the intestine. Calcium has even been added to milk. Consequently, the calcium content of such foods varies according to the manufacturers' policies. Individuals may themselves increase the calcium content of some foods. The addition of vinegar, lemon juice, or even tomatoes to soups, stews, or fish stock that contains bones can increase the calcium content of each cup of liquid. The acid in such items leeches the calcium from the bones during the cooking process. With minimal effort, it is possible to design daily diets containing 1,000–1,500 milligrams of calcium that are low in sodium and cholesterol, taste good, and are not high in calories (see pages 70–73).

Although fruits and vegetables contain calcium, many of them also contain a compound called *oxalic acid*, which binds, or holds, the calcium in the intestine and makes it unavailable to the body. Since spinach, chives, parsley, beet greens, and collards are vegetables that are high in oxalic acid, the absorption of the calcium from these foods is limited. Calcium-containing vegetables that are low in oxalic acid include turnip greens, kale, and endives.

The availability of the calcium in cereals or other foods with a high fiber content likewise depends on the presence of other substances that bind the calcium so that it is not well absorbed. Phytate is such a substance; it is a common ingredient in certain branlike cereals and in unleavened whole wheat products. Meals that contain excessive fat may likewise prevent the absorption of calcium, since fats, like phytate, bind calcium within the intestine.

CALCIUM CONTENT OF FOODS IN THE FOUR ESSENTIAL FOOD GROUPS

MILK-DAIRY GROUP	Calcium milligrams	MEAT AND FISH GROUP	Calcium milligrams
Milks		Alligator meat, 3 oz.	1,055
Skim, 1 cup	301	Bacon, 2 slices	2
2% low-fat, 1 cup	298	Beef, liver, 3 oz.	9
Whole, 1 cup	290	Beef, roast, 3 oz.	10
Powdered, nonfat, dry,		Bologna, 1 oz.	2
1/3 cup	279	Chicken, baked, 3 oz.	13
Buttermilk, 1 cup	284	Egg, large, boiled	29
Evaporated canned,		Frankfurter, 2 oz.	6
1 cup	637	Haddock, fresh, 3 oz.	34
Eggnog, 1 cup	330	Herring, canned, 3 oz.	125
Half-and-half, 1 tbsp.	16	Mackerel, canned,	
		1/2 cup	194
Cheeses		Oysters, canned, 1/2	
American processed,		cup	33
1 oz.	175	Oysters, fresh, 3 oz.	80
Brick, 1 oz.	191	Pork chop, 3 oz.	11
Cheddar, 1 oz.	205	Salmon, with bones,	
Colby, 1 oz.	195	3 oz.	167
Cottage, 1% fat, 1/2 cup	69	Sardines, with bones,	
Edam, 1 oz.	208	3 oz.	372
Monterey Jack, 1 oz.	212	Shrimp, raw, 3 oz.	54
Mozzarella, part skim,		Sole, 3 oz.	61
1 oz.	183	T-bone steak, 3 oz.	8
Parmesan, grated,		Tuna, water-packed,	
1 tbsp.	69	canned, 1/2 cup	14
Ricotta, part skim,		Turkey, 3 oz.	10
1/2 cup	335		
Swiss, 1 oz.	273		
Yogurts, low fat			
Plain, 1 cup	415		
Fruited, 1 cup	345		
Frozen desserts			
Ice milk, 1 cup	176		
Ice cream, 1 cup	176		
Tofu, processed with			
calcium sulfate, 4 oz.	145		

CALCIUM CONTENT OF FOODS
(Continued)

FRUIT-VEGETABLE GROUP	Calcium milligrams	BREAD, NUT, and GRAIN GROUP	Calcium milligrams
Apple, medium	10	**Breads**	
Apricots, dried, 1/2 cup	44	Bagel, 1 whole	9
Asparagus, 1/2 cup	19	Bread, white, 1 slice	21
Banana, medium	4	Bread, whole wheat, 1 slice	23
Beans, green, 1/2 cup	31	Roll, whole wheat	37
Beans, lima, 1/2 cup	31	Crackers, unsalted soda, 6	28
Bok choy, 1/2 cup	126		
Broccoli, 1 stalk	79		
Carrots, 1/2 cup	26		
Corn, 1 medium ear	2	**Cereals**	
Dates, dried, 10	60	All-Bran®, 1 cup	66
Greens, beet, 1/2 cup	72	Cheerios®, 1 cup	32
Greens, collard, 1/2 cup	110	Cornflakes, 1 cup	2
Greens, mustard, 1/2 cup	97	Cream of Wheat®, cooked, 1 cup	6
Greens, turnip, 1/2 cup	133	Oatmeal, cooked, 1 cup	21
Kale, 1/2 cup	103	Raisin bran, 1 cup	26
Orange, medium	54	Rice Krispies®, 1 cup	3
Potato, baked in skin	14	Shredded wheat, 1 cup	17
Spinach, 1/2 cup	116	Total®, 1 cup	40
Tomato, medium	16	Noodles, 1/2 cup	8
Tossed salad	48	Pancake, 6" diameter	157
		Rice, 1/2 cup	10
		Nuts	
		Almonds, 1/2 cup	152
		Brazil nuts, 1/2 cup	130
		Hazel nuts, 1/2 cup	142
		Peanuts, 1/2 cup	50

HIGH-CALCIUM MENU #1

1,553 milligrams Calcium
1,745 Calories
341 milligrams Cholesterol
2,951 milligrams Sodium
18.9+ grams Dietary Fiber

Breakfast	Calcium milligrams	Calories	Cholesterol milligrams	Sodium milligrams	Dietary Fiber grams
2 pancakes, prepared from mix, 6" diameter	314	328	108	824	2.7
2 tsp. margarine	1	67	—*	92	—
2 tbsp. maple syrup	6	96	—	—	—
1/2 cup unsweetened orange juice	12	50	—	1	—
1 cup skim milk	301	86	55	127	—
1 cup decaffeinated coffee	3	2	—	2	—
SUBTOTAL =	637	629	163	1,046	2.7
Lunch					
Grilled tuna and cheese sandwich:					
1/4 cup water-packed tuna	7	54	27	372	—
1 oz. natural cheddar cheese	205	114	30	176	—
2 slices whole wheat bread	46	112	2	242	4.2
1 tsp. margarine	1	34	—	46	—
1 medium fresh pear	13	100	—	3	3.8
3 vanilla wafers	6	54	—	30	—
1 glass iced tea	5	2	—	—	—
SUBTOTAL =	283	470	59	869	8.0
Dinner					
2 1/2" x 2 1/2" x 1 3/4" serving of lasagna	359	374	107	668	1.7
1/2 cup frozen spinach, cooked	116	24	—	53	6.5
1 whole wheat dinner roll	37	90	—	197	unk†
1 tsp. margarine	1	34	—	46	—
2/3 cup ice milk	117	122	12	70	—
1 cup decaffeinated coffee	3	2	—	2	—
SUBTOTAL =	633	646	119	1,036	8.2+
TOTAL =	1,553	1,745	341	2,951	18.9+

*Substance is absent.
†Amount unknown—measurements have not been made.

HIGH-CALCIUM MENU #2

1,524 milligrams Calcium
1,658 Calories
157 milligrams Cholesterol
2,580 milligrams Sodium
15.1+ grams Dietary Fiber

Breakfast	Calcium milligrams	Calories	Cholesterol milligrams	Sodium milligrams	Dietary Fiber grams
1 cup oatmeal	21	156	—*	3	unk†
2 tsp. brown sugar	8	35	—	3	—
2 tbsp. almonds	38	97	—	—	.9
2 tbsp. raisins	11	52	—	5	1.2
1 slice whole wheat toast	23	56	1	121	2.1
1 tsp. margarine	1	34	—	46	—
1 tsp jelly	1	18	—	1	—
1 cup skim milk	301	86	—	127	—
1 cup decaffeinated coffee	3	2	—	2	—
SUBTOTAL =	407	536	1	308	4.2+
Lunch					
Cheese sandwich:					
2 slices whole wheat bread	46	112	2	242	4.2
2 oz. natural cheddar cheese	410	228	60	352	—
10 oz. cream of tomato soup prepared with skim milk	206	161	4	1,170	—
1 medium apple	10	80	—	1	3
1 glass iced tea	5	2	—	—	—
SUBTOTAL =	677	583	66	1,765	7.2
Dinner					
3 1/2 oz. baked chicken breast with skin removed	14	193	82	70	—
1/2 cup brown long grain rice	11	104	—	247	unk
1 tsp. margarine	1	34	—	46	—
1 stalk broccoli	79	23	—	9	3.7
2/3 cup fruited low-fat yogurt with 2 tbsp. nonfat dry milk powder added	332	183	8	133	unk
1 cup decaffeinated coffee	3	2	—	2	—
SUBTOTAL =	440	539	90	507	3.7+
TOTAL =	1,524	1,658	157	2,580	15.1+

*Substance is absent.
†Amount unknown—measurements have not been made.

HIGH-CALCIUM MENU #3

1,014 milligrams Calcium
1,305 Calories
134+ milligrams Cholesterol
1,963 milligrams sodium
18.2+ grams Dietary Fiber

Breakfast	Calcium milligrams	Calories	Cholesterol milligrams	Sodium milligrams	Dietary Fiber grams
1/2 banana	2	51	—*	—	2
1 cup 40% bran flakes cereal	20	132	—	345	6
1 cup skim milk	301	86	5	127	—
1 slice whole wheat toast	23	56	1	121	2.1
1 tsp. margarine	1	34	—	46	—
1 tsp. jelly	1	18	—	1	—
1/2 cup unsweetened orange juice	12	50	—	1	—
1 cup decaffeinated coffee	3	2	—	2	—
SUBTOTAL =	363	429	6	643	10.1
Lunch					
Turkey and Swiss cheese sandwich:					
2 slices whole wheat bread	46	112	2	242	4.2
1 oz. sliced turkey	1	44	15	193	—
1 oz. natural Swiss cheese	273	107	26	74	—
1 tsp. mayonnaise	1	33	3	26	—
1/2 cup fresh fruit cup	15	43	—	1	1.4
2 graham cracker squares	10	119	unk†	204	unk
1 glass iced tea	5	2	—	—	—
SUBTOTAL =	351	460	46+	740	5.6+
Dinner					
4 oz. broiled perch	36	102	66	168	—
1 tbsp. Parmesan cheese	69	23	4	93	—
1/2 cup fresh green beans	31	18	—	4	1.6
1 whole wheat dinner roll	37	90	—	197	unk
1 tsp. margarine	1	34	—	46	—
2/3 cup ice milk	117	122	12	70	—
1/2 cup sliced fresh peaches	6	25	—	1	.9
1 cup decaffeinated coffee	3	2	—	1	—
SUBTOTAL =	300	416	82	580	2.5+
TOTAL =	1,014	1,305	134+	1,963	18.2+

*Substance is absent.
†Amount unknown—measurements have not been made.

HIGH-CALCIUM MENU #4

1,070 milligrams Calcium
1,331 Calories
411+ milligrams Cholesterol
1,847 milligrams sodium
14.5+ grams Dietary Fiber

Breakfast	Calcium milligrams	Calories	Cholesterol milligrams	Sodium milligrams	Dietary Fiber grams
1 scrambled egg made with 2 tbsp. skim milk	67	90	280	86	—*
2 slices whole wheat toast	46	112	2	242	4.2
2 tsp. margarine	1	67	—	92	—
2 tsp. jelly	2	36	—	2	—
1/2 grapefruit	16	40	—	1	.6
1 cup skim milk	301	86	5	127	—
1 cup decaffeinated coffee	3	2	—	2	—
SUBTOTAL =	436	433	287	552	4.8
Lunch					
1/2 cup cottage cheese, 1% fat	69	81	5	459	—
6 unsalted soda crackers	28	70	unk†	120	unk
1 cup fresh strawberries	32	56	—	2	3.4
1 tomato, sliced	16	27	—	4	2.5
2 oatmeal raisin cookies	16	108	10	82	.3
1 glass iced tea	5	2	—	—	—
SUBTOTAL =	166	344	15+	667	6.2+
Dinner					
Cheeseburger					
1 oz. natural cheddar cheese	205	114	30	176	—
3 oz. lean ground beef patty	11	161	77	51	—
1 hamburger bun	30	119	—	202	1.2
1/2 cup carrots	26	24	—	26	2.3
1/2 cup chocolate pudding made with skim milk	193	134	2	172	—
1 cup decaffeinated coffee	3	2	—	1	—
SUBTOTAL =	468	554	109	628	3.5
TOTAL =	1,070	1,331	411+	1,847	14.5+

*Substance is absent.
†Amount unknown—measurements have not been made.

HIGH-SODIUM CEREALS

Cereal	Sodium per serving in milligrams
Ready-to-eat cereals:	
Cheerios® (General Mills)	290
Kix® (General Mills)	290
Rice Krispies® (Kellogg's)	290
Corn Flakes (Kellogg's)	290
Bran Chex® (Ralston)	300
Corn Chex® (Ralston)	310
Product 19® (Kellogg's)	320
Wheaties® (General Mills)	370
Hot cereals:	
Cream of Wheat®, instant, original flavor (Nabisco)	180
Cream of Wheat®, instant, various flavors (Nabisco)	180–240
Oatmeal, instant, various flavors (Quaker Oats)	135–360
Corn Grits, instant, regular flavor (Quaker Oats)	440
Corn Grits, instant, country bacon flavor (Quaker Oats)	590

A low salt, or sodium, content, of course, is as desirable as a high calcium content for most people, and the sodium content in many foods is surprisingly high. Some of the commonly used cereals, for example, have more sodium than an equivalent serving of potato chips, corn chips, or cheese snacks! Although many East Asian foods contain a significant amount of calcium—in particular, seaweeds (wakame, hijiki, tangle, and nori), bok choy, sesame seeds, almonds, sweetfish, tofu, and natto—some, such as oriental-style frozen vegetables and miso soy products also contain high amounts of sodium. One must also consider the fact that the average sodium content of a 1–1½ cup serving of an East Asian dish seasoned with soy sauce or teriyaki sauce or processed with monosodium glutamate is 1,000 milligrams! Monosodium glutamate contains no calcium but does contain 615 milligrams of sodium per teaspoon. Sodium content of soy sauce or teriyaki sauce is 343 and 230 milligrams per teaspoon, respectively. Many East Asian foods also contain a large amount of oxalic acid in oriental vegetables, which could also limit the calcium benefit of such foods.

An important message for children and grandchildren: A good supply of calcium is required for bones to grow and mature fully and to become as strong as possible. Bone tissue losses that may be related to calcium begin early in life and continue to the maturity of bone and beyond—long after the body has stopped growing taller.

CALCIUM AND REDUCTION IN BONE LOSS IN POSTMENOPAUSAL WOMEN

Not all scientists agree that increasing calcium intake to 1,000–1,500 milligrams daily will prevent osteoporosis. There is agreement that a high calcium intake is needed during adolescence to build the strongest possible bones (another message for your children and grandchildren). Furthermore, evidence is substantial that a high calcium intake reduces bone loss after age sixty. On the other hand, a newly menopausal woman at high risk for osteoporosis should certainly not rely on calcium alone to protect her and should consider also that whatever effect calcium does have in suppressing bone loss may be greater in those women who have had a deficiency of calcium in their diet for most of their lives. A high calcium intake will not be as effective as estrogen therapy (ET) in diminishing the rapid bone loss that occurs during the five to ten years after menopause (see chapter 11). However, an adequate supply of calcium may aid in attaining a favorable response to ET and to other methods for reducing bone loss, including calcitonin therapy and physical exercise.

Recently, the mineral boron, found in some fruits and vegetables, has been reported in one study to reduce calcium losses in the urine and to increase the amount of estrogen in the blood. More information is needed to confirm this finding and to determine whether boron, previously not thought essential for good health, helps prevent bone loss. Boron is toxic when taken in large amounts.

SIDE EFFECTS OF INCREASED CALCIUM CONSUMPTION

Excessive calcium consumption—brought about by increasing dietary calcium, taking calcium supplements, or both—may be associated with certain side effects. These are discussed in the following paragraphs; calcium supplements in general are discussed in the next chapter. At the intake recommended by a U.S. government-sponsored panel that convened to analyze the preventive approach for osteoporosis (1,000-1,500 milligrams per day), no complications can be expected. Although some may worry about the effect of calcium supplements on the blood calcium level, calcium supplements in doses of 1,000-1,500 milligrams per day are not a cause for concern. Doses higher than 2,500 milligrams per day may raise the blood and urine calcium. The problem of kidney stones occurring when calcium supplements are ingested in doses of 1,000-1,500 milligrams per day has been overemphasized.

Nevertheless, there are situations in which one should not increase one's calcium intake, either through diet or calcium supplements, without a physician's advice. *A history of kidney stones or kidney infections, a family history of kidney stones, or any current medical illness* demands a doctor's recommendation. Some patients with kidney stones have high levels of calcium in their blood and urine because they absorb too much calcium from their diet or release too much calcium from their bones through excessive bone resorption. Among the conditions that can cause these problems are hyperparathyroidism, certain types of cancer (such as multiple myeloma), an overactive thyroid (or the presence of too much thyroid medication in the system), sarcoidosis (a disease that mainly affects the lungs, lymph nodes, liver, and eyes), and tuberculosis.

**AVERAGE DAILY ENERGY AND ZINC INTAKES
OF ELDERLY PARTICIPANTS IN NATIONAL SURVEY***

Group	Age	Energy (calories)	Zinc (milligrams)
Men	65–74	1,970	10.5
	75+	1,808	9.3
Women	65–74	1,444	7.6
	75+	1,367	7.0

*Based on data from Sandstead et al, *American Journal of Clinical Nutrition* 36: 1046, 1982.

**UNITED STATES RECOMMENDED DAILY ALLOWANCES
(USRDA) FOR MINERALS***

	Age years	Calcium milligrams	Phosphorus milligrams	Magnesium milligrams	Iron milligrams	Zinc milligrams
Infants	birth–12 months	600	500	70	15	5
Children	under 4 years	800	800	200	10	8
Adults and Children	4 or more years	1,000	1,000	400	18	15
Pregnant or Lactating Women		1,300	1,300	450	18	15

*The USRDAs are nutrient standards set by the Food and Drug Administration in 1973 using the Recommended Dietary Allowances of the National Academy of Sciences, National Research Council. The USRDAs are established for four age-sex groups. Generally, the highest values in the RDA table were selected for use within each USRDA category. The nutritional information on food labels is expressed as percent of the USRDA.

Modified from information presented in the FDA consumer memo, *Nutrition Labels and U.S. RDA,* publication 81-2146, U.S. Government Printing Office, Washington, D.C., 1981.

RECOMMENDED DIETARY ALLOWANCES OF MINERALS PER DAY*

Food and Nutrition Board, National Academy of Sciences
National Research Council

Designed for the maintenance of good nutrition
of practically all healthy people in the USA

	Age years	Calcium milligrams	Phosphorus milligrams	Magnesium milligrams	Iron milligrams	Zinc milligrams
Infants	0.0–0.5	360	240	50	10	3
	0.5–1.0	540	360	70	15	5
Children	1–3	800	800	150	15	10
	4–6	800	800	200	10	10
	7–10	800	800	250	10	10
Males	11–14	1,200	1,200	350	18	15
	15–18	1,200	1,200	400	18	15
	19–22	800	800	350	10	15
	23–50	800	800	350	10	15
	51+	800	800	350	10	15
Females	11–14	1,200	1,200	300	18	15
	15–18	1,200	1,200	300	18	15
	19–22	800	800	300	18	15
	23–50	800	800	300	18	15
	51+	800	800	300	10	15
Pregnant		+400	+400	+150	†	+5
Lactating		+400	+400	+150	†	+10

* Modified from National Research Council: *Recommended Dietary Allowances.* Ninth edition. Washington, D.C., National Academy of Sciences, 1980.
    The allowances are intended to provide for individual variations among most normal persons as they live in the United States under usual environmental stresses. Diets should be based on a variety of common foods in order to provide other nutrients for which human requirements have been less well defined.

† Pregnant and lactating women cannot ingest enough iron in their diets and must take iron supplements.

There is no need to take more than 1,500 milligrams of calcium a day as a total intake. Calcium intakes of 3,000–5,000 milligrams a day may stimulate the binding of phytate to other essential substances such as zinc, thus preventing absorption of zinc from the intestine and causing deficiency of that essential element. (Certain water pills and chronic alcohol abuse will also deplete the body of zinc.) Zinc deficiency, which may lead to alterations in the sense of taste and poor wound healing, is a particular problem in the elderly. The results of a recent National Food Consumption Survey by the U.S. Department of Agriculture show that elderly population groups consume about one-half to two-thirds of the zinc RDA.

The current RDA and USRDA for zinc is 15 milligrams. This can be achieved by a generally balanced and nutritionally adequate diet that contains shellfish, dark poultry meat, and red meats. *Zinc supplements should not be taken in any form without a physician's advice.* If they are added to the diet, the supplement should be no greater than 15-40 milligrams per day. Too much zinc can cause anemia.

There are also claims that the use of calcium supplements interferes with magnesium absorption. Careful studies in adults do not substantiate these claims. Calcium intakes of 1,000–1,500 milligrams daily are not likely to promote magnesium loss in healthy individuals. Moreover, magnesium intakes above the USRDA for magnesium of 400 milligrams per day (in nonpregnant adults) do not decrease the need for the appropriate amount of calcium.

Since magnesium deficiency is rare, there is no need to supplement diets with magnesium. Chronic alcohol or diuretic abuse can result in magnesium deficiency, as can diabetic conditions that are not well controlled (associated with repeated occurrences of an accumulation of acids in the bloodstream and with high blood sugar levels). Theoretically, anyone who eats a diet containing an abundance of processed or refined foods can become magnesium-deficient, since these modern refinements remove magnesium. Magnesium is contained in high concentrations in green vegetables and seafood, as well as in milk, nuts, and whole grains.

HARMFUL EFFECTS OF EXCESS OF VITAMIN D

Excessive vitamin D intake (greater than 400–1,200 International Units [IU] per day) should also be avoided, since overdosage with vitamin D will result in a rise in blood calcium and the amount of calcium excreted in the urine. The FDA has not set upper limits on allowable levels of vitamins in products sold over the counter. There is surely no harm in taking an over-the-counter vitamin D preparation that contains no more than the RDA or USRDA (400 IU per day), as is found in some calcium supplement preparations. The routine use of large amounts, or megadoses, of vitamin D—which is a common practice for vitamins A, E, and C—is impractical and dangerous. (A megadose is defined as a dose of a vitamin or mineral that is ten times the RDA.) Not only does the body not require such large doses but also excessive vitamin D intake may cause serious side effects such as kidney stones and a rise in the blood calcium. Symptoms of this condition include fatigue, intestinal upset, changes in personality, and headaches. Elderly people who develop even a small elevation in blood calcium may actually have mental problems that resemble Alzheimer's disease. One should choose vitamin D supplements cautiously, making sure that the supplement does not contain a megadose.

The need for vitamin D supplementation will depend on certain habits, such as the extent of routine sunlight exposure, the type of drugs that are prescribed for specific health problems, and the presence of skin disorders that require decreased sunlight exposure. As little as thirty minutes of direct exposure to sunlight daily will ensure adequate vitamin D production in the skin. But the harmful consequences of sunlight, such as skin cancers, are a concern. The diet is a safe source of vitamin D. High-dose supplements are not needed unless there is a medical indication and should not be taken without a physician's advice. If taking vitamin D supplements, one should remember the following:

- For people who are taking no drugs and who may have limited sunlight exposure because they don't get outdoors routinely, 400 IU of vitamin D daily should be sufficient to prevent vitamin D deficiency. There is some evidence that people over the age of sixty-five may need more, perhaps 800–1,200 IU—not a megadose—but a physican's advice should be obtained.

- The use of drugs such as corticosteroids and those used to treat epilepsy or changes in heartbeats (Dilantin®) or the presence of osteomalacia may require an individual to take more vitamin D than the RDA. In this case, a physician will obtain a blood test for vitamin D content and prescribe the necessary dosage.

BENEFICIAL EFFECT OF CALCIUM WITH CANCER AND HIGH BLOOD PRESSURE

It has been suggested but not proven that men with lower dietary levels of calcium have a higher risk of getting cancer of the colon (large intestine) and rectum. In one study, calcium supplements of 1,250 milligrams (as calcium carbonate) a day decreased the growth rate of intestinal cells obtained from people with a family history of cancer of the colon. Further research is needed to determine whether doses of calcium recommended to maintain bone health could also be helpful for those individuals with a tendency to develop cancer of the colon.

There is some evidence that an adequate intake of calcium may be beneficial for some people with high blood pressure, or hypertension. Calcium supplementation has been given to lower blood pressure in some pregnant women with hypertension and in other patients (both men and women) with mild hypertension who are receiving other blood pressure lowering drugs. This is also an area where more research is needed.

9 • Calcium Supplements

Although a well-selected and appropriate diet can offer sufficient calcium to maintain bone health, this approach may be impractical, since individuals may be unable to adjust their diets according to their needs—either because this involves altering eating styles or because of food intolerances. It may also be tedious to plan on a daily basis meals that contain the required amount of calcium. Moreover, not only must the foods be adjusted to maximize the *availability* of the calcium ingested, but they also should be selected to contain enough calcium to counteract the effects of drugs on calcium absorption by the intestine and excretion in the urine. For example, individuals who are taking either thyroid hormone preparations or cortisone-like drugs need more calcium than recommended, since these drugs decrease the absorption of calcium and increase calcium loss in the urine.

A variety of calcium preparations are now available to supplement the daily dietary intake. To find out whether a supplement is needed, and, if so, how much, one should first estimate one's usual dietary intake of calcium. Remember that a diet deficient of milk or cheese will contain only about 200–300 milligrams of calcium if calcium-supplemented foods are not being used. To guarantee an intake of 1,000–1,500 milligrams of calcium per day without dairy products or calcium-supplemented foods, an additional 700–1,200 milligrams of calcium is required. To reach this quota, choose the calcium supplement that delivers a large amount of elemental calcium per pill. Elemental calcium is the actual amount of calcium in the supplement. All supplements contain calcium as part of a salt—calcium carbonate, calcium citrate, calcium gluconate, calcium phosphate—much like sodium in sodium chloride, or table salt. The calcium in some supplements is absorbed as well as calcium in milk. Calcium in some supplements—for example, in calcium phosphate—is not as biologically available as in other supplements. Some supplements are labeled with the amount of calcium salt, which is always much greater than the amount of elemental calcium. To ensure the needed amount of elemental calcium, it is prudent to select a calcium supplement that contains the largest amount of calcium per pill (see page 84). That is why calcium carbonate preparations are often recommended. One or two tablets of calcium carbonate per day, each of which contains 500 or 600 milligrams of calcium, may be all that you need! One should be sure to select the dose based on the amount of *elemental* calcium in the preparation.

Regarding calcium supplements, remember the following:

- With limited exceptions, calcium carbonate must be taken with meals or no later than one to one-and-a-half hours later to ensure maximum absorption. Stomach acid stimulated by the meal is needed to dissolve the calcium, and many older people do not produce enough stomach acid between meals.

- Do not take more than 500 or 600 milligrams of calcium at one time. If more is needed, take it in separate doses at different meals—for example, with breakfast and dinner. Total daily intake of calcium (through diet and/or supplements) should not exceed 1,500 milligrams.

- Beware of dolomite and bonemeal calcium carbonate preparations, since they may contain excessive amounts of potentially poisonous substances such as lead. Although some antacids (TUMS® and Titralac®, for example) are sources of calcium carbonate, antacids that

GENERAL DOSING INFORMATION FOR CALCIUM SUPPLEMENTS

The action of calcium supplements depends upon their calcium content. Various calcium supplements contain different amounts of elemental calcium by weight.

Calcium Supplement	% elemental calcium by weight
Calcium Carbonate	40
Calcium Chloride	27.2
Calcium Citrate	21.1
Calcium Glubionate*	6.5
Calcium Gluceptate	8.2
Calcium Gluconate	9
Calcium Lactate	13
Calcium Phosphate	
Dibasic	23
Tribasic	38

* Available in syrup form.

contain sodium bicarbonate, aluminum hydroxide, or magnesium hydroxide are not effective calcium supplements and should not be used for this purpose.

- Be wary of generic forms of calcium supplements, since many do not dissolve well or do not release the calcium in the stomach. Lists of commercial calcium supplements that are not recommended are now available to physicians and pharmacists. Consult your doctor or pharmacist for advice.

- Do not take calcium carbonate (or sodium bicarbonate) together with iron supplements, since the absorption of the iron may be decreased. When calcium carbonate and iron supplements are in the same tablet, the absorption of the iron will be normal if the tablet also contains vitamin C. Liquid antacids containing aluminum hydroxide and magnesium hydroxide do not decrease iron absorption but do not, of course, supply calcium.

- Avoid taking the calcium supplement with certain foods such as rhubarb, red meat, bread, cola drinks, bran, spinach, and whole-grain cereals. These foods contain chemicals that combine with calcium, so the calcium is not "free" to be absorbed as pure, or elemental, calcium.
- Avoid excessive use of alcoholic beverages, tobacco, or caffeine-containing beverages.
- Constipation occasionally caused by unabsorbed calcium carbonate may be decreased by taking the calcium carbonate with meals and drinking more water during the day, especially in the hot weather.
- Don't take supplements within one to two hours of taking any other medicine by mouth. They may decrease the absorption of the medicine.
- High zinc intake, greater than 140 milligrams per day, decreases calcium absorption if calcium intake is low but not if calcium intake is as recommended.

The possible side effects of excessive calcium ingestion are discussed in chapter 8. Following the above guidelines however, will in most cases ensure that side effects do not develop.

10 • *Physical Exercise and Bone Health*

Physical exercise, combined with proper nutrition, helps maintain wellness and a pleasant body image and increases the ability to cope with life stresses by improving mental outlook. A routine exercise program can also do the following:

- Allow the heart to handle sudden demands for increased work, as when shoveling snow, running to catch a bus or airplane, or just climbing stairs rapidly.
- Decrease body fat.
- Increase muscle tone, strength, and endurance. Improved strength can help prevent fractures by reducing the chances of falling or decreasing the severity of injury caused by a fall.
- Aid in controlling blood pressure; some people who must take drugs for high blood pressure may require less medication if they exercise regularly.
- Improve the control of blood sugar in patients with diabetes mellitus; often exercise will allow a decrease in the dose of insulin or oral drugs.

- Reduce the tendency for blood fats and cholesterol to accumulate in plaques on artery walls (atherosclerosis); this may help prevent heart attack.
- Reduce depression and anxiety while promoting a feeling of well-being.
- Decrease the formation of dangerous internal blood clots because of increased blood flow and the production of substances in the body that prevent rapid blood clotting.

EXERCISE AND BONE ACCUMULATION

Although not all the scientific evidence is in, there is reason to believe that physical exercise can increase the accumulation of bone. People who have lost the function of their arms or legs, either because of an accident or a stroke, rapidly lose bone tissue. The more active the muscle covering a bone, the stronger the bone seems to become. Just look at the arms of a professional tennis or jai alai player. The amount of muscle is greater in the arm used to hold the racket. The racket arm also has heavier bones, more bone tissue. On the other hand, prolonged space flight, which reduces the effect of muscles on the skeleton, causes loss of bone tissue.

Two main kinds of studies have addressed the possible impact of exercise on bone mass: cross-sectional studies (looking at subjects "after the fact"), which compare bone mass in individuals who have exercised and those who have not, and "prospective studies," which examine the effect of planned exercise programs on subsequent changes in bone. In cross-sectional studies, young healthy female marathon runners with normal menstrual periods have more bone than inactive women of the same age and sex. Recently, the same pattern was found in healthy long-distance runners of both sexes who began running after age fifty.

Evidence that a routine exercise program may reduce bone loss in persons who have osteoporosis is now available from studies designed to measure bone mass before and after planned exercise routines such as walking; running; programmed ball games; standing, sitting, and lying exercises; and more vigorous programs involving either treadmill or indoor track running for periods of eight months to three years. In all instances these weight-bearing (working against the pull of gravity) exercises appeared to decrease the rate of bone loss in those people who performed them faithfully at least three times a week for periods of thirty to forty-five minutes. In fact, the amount of bone was reported to increase in many women. (Moderate swimming and bicycling programs have not been studied as extensively as other forms of exercise; not strictly weight-bearing, they may not emerge as beneficial for retaining bone tissue.) Thus, good exercise habits may promote bone health. Combined with good nutritional habits and, if indicated, appropriate therapy, exercise may well be beneficial to the individual with osteoporosis. Since exercise is not a proven preventive or cure, it is particularly important that individuals select an exercise program that is convenient and safe. There is no place for indiscriminate exercise. The following paragraphs suggest a reasonable approach.

SPECIFIC FORMS OF EXERCISE

There are two general kinds of exercise programs: (1) *aerobic or isotonic exercises,* which increase the heart rate and improve the body's use of oxygen by the rhythmic movement of large muscle groups for a long period of time, and (2) *isometric exercises,* which increase muscle strength but have little effect on the heart or oxygen use. Examples of aerobic exercises are jogging, swimming, cross-country skiing, cycling, tennis, handball, and dancing. Walking is also an aerobic exercise, as long as it is brisk and uses the large muscles in the lower body and appropriate arm-swinging movements. Isometric exercises include pull-ups, leg and arm lifts, weight lifting, hand grips, and push-ups. Although both forms of exercise may be helpful, strenuous isometric exercises are of limited value, since they can actually raise blood pressure and do not appear to help the heart.

OBTAINING THE MAXIMAL BENEFIT FROM AEROBIC EXERCISE

Although an exercise program can begin with a variety of activities, it is important to prepare by warming up for five to ten minutes. This is usually done by simple stretches (avoid extreme stretching), deep breathing, or jogging in place slowly. Some physical therapists advocate stretching only later in the warm-up period, to decrease the likelihood of muscle and tendon injury. The level of activity should increase gradually over days and weeks, especially in elderly people or those who have not been in the exercise habit. In the beginning, exercise periods of fifteen to twenty minutes are sufficient to produce the desired effects on the heart, lungs, and muscles, provided that an appropriate target heart rate—heartbeats per minute—is achieved. The heart rate, or pulse, gauges the impact of the exercise on the heart and therefore its potential benefit. The target pulse is what the pulse should be in order to realize the maximal benefit from aerobic exercise. The target pulse depends on one's age and maximum *predicted pulse;* maximum predicted pulse is 220 minus age in years (150 for a seventy-year-old person). To determine the target pulse, the maximum pulse is multiplied by 0.70 and 0.80. For example, for the seventy-year-old person, with the maximum predicted pulse of 150 beats per minute, the target pulse is between 0.70 × 150 (which equals 105) and 0.80 × 150 (which equals 120). Thus, when exercising, a seventy-year-old person should aim for a pulse of between 105 and 120. One can determine the pulse by feeling the artery at the wrist with the fingertips of the other hand. It is best to begin exercising slowly and to reach the target pulse gradually, maintaining it for fifteen to twenty minutes. Later on, when the body has adjusted to the need for additional effort, the exercise period can be extended to thirty to forty-five minutes. Strenuous exercises should be followed by a cooling-off period with a gradual decrease in the activity over a period of five minutes.

How often one exercises is a matter of individual life pattern and time commitment. Periods of aerobic exercise

UPRIGHT EXERCISES
(Several times a day.)

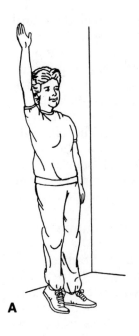
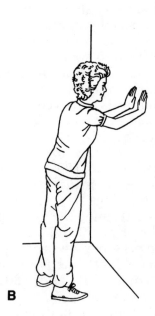

A. Flatten your body against a wall. Stretch as high as possible, lifting your right heel while extending your right arm above your head and keeping your back flat. Alternate with the left hand. Do five time.

B. Stand facing a wall with your feet twelve to sixteen inches from the base of the wall. Place your hands on the wall at eye height. Push against the wall while keeping your back straight. Hold for a count of five. Repeat ten times.

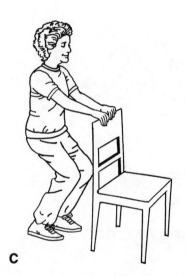 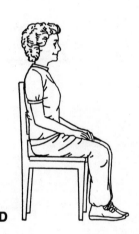

C.   D.

C. Stand in back of a sturdy chair with your feet twelve inches from the back legs. Bend your knees and lower your back as far as is comfortable for you, keeping your back straight at all times. Do five times.

D. Sit in a sturdy wooden or metal chair with a straight back. Place your back firmly against the back of the chair. Hold for a count of five. Repeat ten times.

RECLINING EXERCISES
(Twice daily, five to ten times each.)

These exercises can be performed while lying on the floor or on a firm mattress.

A

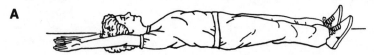

B

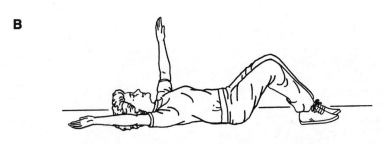

C

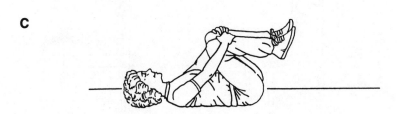

A. Extend both arms and legs as far as possible while keeping your back flat and in a straight position. Hold for a count of five. Repeat ten times.

B. Bend both knees. Keeping your back straight, raise and stretch your left arm overhead, pressing your shoulder into the floor or support mattress. Do ten times. Repeat with your right arm.

C. Pull both knees up, using both hands, and bring them close to your chest, stretching your lower back. Hold to a count of five. Repeat ten times.

D

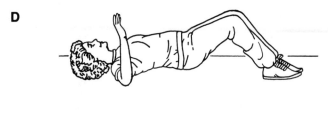

E

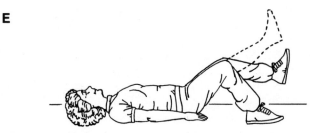

F

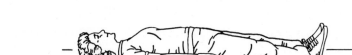

D. With knees bent and elbows in a horizontal position, press your elbows into the floor or support mattress. Hold for a count of five. Repeat ten times.

E. Bend your knees, keeping your back straight. Raise your left knee as high as it will go. Do five times. Repeat with the right knee.

F. Keep your back flat and your arms and hands at your sides. Contract your back muscles, buttocks, and thighs. Hold for a count of five. Repeat ten times.

as infrequent as three days a week do strengthen the heart and body muscles. And remember, even a good walking exercise program can burn calories and keep you slim. Whatever exercise is used, consistency and routine are important. Lack of exercise for three to four months can dissipate all the benefit of the previous exercise.

PRACTICAL EXERCISES FOR OLDER INDIVIDUALS

Before starting an exercise program, one must consider the available facilities, one's individual endurance potential, the amount of pleasure one will gain from exercise, physical limitations, and general health status.

Once these factors are evaluated and analyzed, the type of exercise and the nature of the program can be designed. An exercise program should be one that can be performed routinely and that is not so difficult, time-consuming, and tedious that routine performance becomes a chore. Individuals who have osteoporosis and weakened spines should restrict themselves to programs offering exercises that require only standing, sitting, or reclining. Exercises that actually flex the spine, such as strenuous sit-ups and toe touches, should be avoided. These exercises can actually produce new spinal fractures or worsen existing fractures.

Walking is excellent exercise. As noted by Jeannie Ralston in *Walking for the Health of It* (Washington, D.C.: AARP; Glenview, Ill.: Scott, Foresman & Co., 1985), it is easy and effective for people over fifty. It strengthens both the back and stomach muscles. Programmed walks four times a week beginning with periods of ten to twenty minutes at the appropriate heart rate improve heart and muscle function, relieve depression, and aid in concentrating. One should start slowly the first week, attempting to walk one mile in twenty minutes four times a week, increasing gradually so that in three months, one is walking three miles in forty-five minutes four times a week.

Since between 1,500 and 2,000 steps may be taken during a mile walk, feet should be checked for corns, calluses, bunions, and blisters. Correct, properly fitted shoes with good heel supports are essential, and socks should be used that have a high percentage of cotton or wool, since they will help absorb the perspiration and protect the insides of the shoes. Socks made of synthetic fibers and nylon will increase foot perspiration. Diabetics must be especially careful to examine their feet before and after each walk for blisters, irritations (redness), and early infections. Some diabetics have numb feet and can be seriously injured by ill-fitting shoes or foreign objects in the shoes, which they cannot feel.

The appropriate and planned use of leisure time for activities such as gardening, golfing, or even climbing stairs can also suffice as exercise regimens if these activities are performed in an established routine fashion and are incorporated into the daily routine.

Remember, strenuous exercises can be harmful. They can lead to muscular or skeletal injury, provoke heart attack or a disturbance in heart rhythm, and raise blood pressure. Individuals forty and older should have a thorough medical examination before embarking on an aerobic exercise program and must obtain the advice of their physician about the type, frequency, and duration of exercise. (Younger individuals with any illness or receiving any drugs should not begin such a program without a physician's advice.) Individuals who are at high risk for heart disease may need to have a stress test before initiating an exercise program. A stress test can disclose possible danger of strenuous exercise to the heart. Even moderate physical exercise may prove harmful when excessive sweating occurs without necessary fluid intake. Dehydration may lead to the formation of either uric acid or calcium oxalate crystals in urine and increase the risk of kidney stone formation.

11 • *Estrogen Therapy (ET) After Menopause*

A woman entering the menopausal years today can expect to live more than thirty additional years. She will spend more than one-third of her life with lowered levels of estrogen than she had when she was younger. This reduction in estrogen causes two major changes in a woman's health: disturbing symptoms of varying degrees and bone tissue loss. A third change, susceptibility to heart attack, may also be related to estrogen reduction.

DISTURBING SYMPTOMS

As many as nine out of ten postmenopausal women will experience some distressing symptoms. Due mainly to lowered estrogen levels, symptoms include hot flushes (usually brief periods of warmth and a reddening or blushing of the skin), hot flashes (episodes of warmth with no skin blushing), sweating episodes with the flushes and flashes, insomnia, depression, other mood and personality changes, voice change, dizziness, aching muscles and joints, back pain, and breast shrinkage. In addition, drying of the vaginal tissues and of the lower urinary passages can make intercourse difficult and painful; cause itching and bleeding; result in a burning sensation while urinating, a sense of urgency to urinate, and more frequent urination; and increase the likelihood of vaginal and urinary tract infections. Weakened pelvic tissues predispose to a prolapse (protrusion) of the uterus from the vagina.

It is the hot flush or flash that most women equate with the disturbing symptoms of menopause. Most postmenopausal women will experience these sudden feelings of warmth and reddening at the chest, neck, face, and arms that last, on average, about three minutes and are often accompanied by sweating. Many women will experience them several years before the last menstrual period, and they can still occur five to ten years afterward. Not uncommonly, sleep is disturbed by these episodes, and loss of sleep can cause daytime fatigue and anxiety. Although lowered estrogen levels are responsible for these symptoms and estrogen therapy eliminates them, the actual changes in the body's chemistry that trigger them are not well understood. The brain, affected by loss of estrogens, appears to mastermind other chemical changes in the body that cause hot flushes and flashes.

BONE LOSS

Menopausal decreases in estrogen speed up bone loss. Whereas premenopausal women over the age of thirty

---

DISTURBING SYMPTOMS OF MENOPAUSE

Hot "Flushes" and "Flashes"
Sweating Episodes
Painful Intercourse—Vaginal Dryness
Painful Urination
Urgent, Frequent Need to Urinate
Itching of the Vagina
Breast Shrinkage
Aching in Muscles and Joints
Backache
Headache
Insomnia
Depression and Other Personality Changes

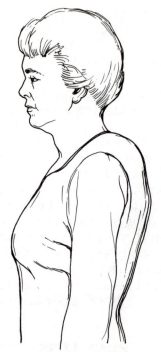

**Woman with Hunched Back
Often Occurring with Osteoporosis**

may lose less than 1 percent of their bone tissue yearly, losses not uncommonly reach 3 percent per year for the five to ten years that follow the menopause. Loss of bone tissue from the spine is particularly dramatic during this period; consequently, postmenopausal women with osteoporosis are at special risk for crush fractures of the vertebrae.

HEART DISEASE

Menopause also appears to end the relative protection from heart disease enjoyed by younger women. Premenopausal women are less likely than men of the same age to develop coronary atherosclerosis—narrowing of the arteries to the heart (coronary arteries) by cholesterol-filled plaques. They are not as likely as men to suffer from heart attack. Evidence suggests that after menopause women are no longer protected; the incidence of heart attack rises. A significant postmenopausal change in blood cholesterol may be the culprit.

Cholesterol in the blood combines with complex chemicals called lipoproteins; one family of such chemicals, high-density lipoproteins (HDL), has been shown to reduce the risk of atherosclerosis, while another family, low-density lipoproteins (LDL), increases risk. After menopause, LDL-cholesterol tends to rise and HDL-cholesterol to fall, thus setting the stage for acceleration of atherosclerosis. Of course, menopause, with its changes in blood cholesterol, is just one of many factors influencing the risk of heart disease, including heredity, diet, blood pressure, cigarette smoking, and the presence of disorders such as diabetes mellitus.

ESTROGEN ADMINISTRATION

Because decreased estrogen appears to underlie the disturbing symptoms as well as the susceptibility to bone loss experienced by postmenopausal women, it is not surprising that scientists have studied the ability of estrogen administration to blunt or relieve those problems. Estrogen preparations, both natural (derived from tissues and fluids) and synthetic, have been available for decades. Estrogen therapy (ET) eases most menopausal effects: hot flushes, sweating, and discomfort caused by drying and shrinkage of the vagina and lower urinary tract. Just relief of those symptoms can make a woman feel better—improve her sense of well-being and therefore her outlook on life. It is not known definitely whether estrogens relieve insomnia, aches, pains, and personality changes, but doctors have the impression that they do, at least in *some* women.

Many studies have been done to determine whether estrogens protect the postmenopausal woman against heart attack and other kinds of vascular accidents. Unfortunately, proof that ET has such an effect is still not available. A protective effect, though unproven, seems likely from most available evidence; more studies are needed to establish this effect without a doubt. ET does tend to restore blood cholesterol levels back to where they were before menopause—the "good" cholesterol (HDL) rises, and the "bad" cholesterol (LDL) falls. Some studies suggest that estrogens protect against heart attack in other ways, perhaps by a beneficial effect on the arteries. There should be a decreased incidence of heart attack, judging from these changes. That decrease has not been proven, however, and because of uncertainty about possible benefit to the heart, ET cannot yet be advocated for this purpose alone.

REDUCTION IN BONE LOSS

ET in pill form reduces the loss of bone tissue in postmenopausal women. Oral estrogen is approved by the Food and Drug Administration (FDA) for treating osteoporosis. Estrogens have been shown to diminish the decline in bone mass—as measured by SPA, DPA, and CAT—at many sites throughout the skeleton, including the vertebrae, wrist, hip, and other bones. Some studies have shown an actual elimination of bone loss in estrogen-treated women after menopause, just at a stage in life when they are losing bone tissue most rapidly. Prevention of bone loss is important only if it ultimately preserves bone strength and reduces fracture risk. Since bone mass is what determines bone strength, one might have anticipated that preserving bone mass tends to prevent fracture. Numerous studies have indeed indicated that estrogen-treated postmenopausal women are less likely to break a bone than untreated women. It has been estimated that ET for five years after the menopause would decrease by 50 percent a woman's chances of having a hip fracture later in life. This projection emphasizes that ET works best when bone loss is fastest, during the first five to ten years after menopause. In a woman at high risk for osteoporosis, it follows that ET should be started as soon after the menopause as possible. Estrogen also slows the more gradual bone loss that occurs after age sixty to sixty-five, but starting ET long after the menopause cannot be expected to decrease fracture risk as much as earlier therapy, since much bone has already been lost, and estrogen will not bring about the repair of a deficient skeleton. When ET is stopped, bone loss resumes. But postponing bone loss for five to ten years or more means a stronger skeleton later on. Thus, ET is an investment in bone health—it has long-lasting benefits.

ET CONTROVERSY

ET is the most effective way to relieve disturbing menopausal symptoms and to prevent osteoporosis, yet it has been a controversial topic. Until recently, many women were reluctant to accept ET, fearful of its complications. To be sure, there are circumstances under which ET cannot be used. These include the presence or suspicion of certain cancers, such as some types of breast cancer and cancer of the endometrium, that depend on estrogen for growth; a previously experienced significant complication of ET; current problems with blood clots in the arteries or veins; and unexplained vaginal bleeding. In addition, ET is not generally recommended for a woman with a blood relative who has had breast cancer. A small percentage of noncancerous breast lumps (fibrocystic disease) contain precancerous lesions; this condition should be evaluated before ET is instituted. ET may worsen several conditions, including otosclerosis, and uncommon, often hereditary cause of hearing loss; fibroid tumor of the uterus; and porphyria, a very rare disorder in which blood pigments accumulate in the body and cause symptoms such as severe stomach pain and headache. Pregnancy is a contraindication for premenopausal women.

There are other situations, not strictly contraindications, in which ET is not generally recommended, such as the presence of gallbladder disease. This and other problems—including diabetes mellitus, hypertension, and a propensity to form blood clots—were discovered in younger women who were taking high doses of estrogen as part of the birth control pill. Doctors do not really know how often they will occur in postmenopausal women taking the low doses of estrogen that are recommended to prevent osteoporosis. There is evidence that low-dose ET

BENEFITS OF ET

- Reduces or eliminates disturbing menopausal symptoms.
- Reduces bone loss and thus prevents fractures.
- May protect against heart attack.

CONTRAINDICATIONS TO ET

Known or suspected cancer that needs estrogen to grow.
Complication of ET in the past.
Undiagnosed vaginal bleeding.
Blood clots in arteries or veins.
Unwillingness to have medical checkups.
Pregnancy, for premenopausal women.

---

actually lowers blood pressure in some postmenopausal women and has no major effects on blood clotting. Another important fact has emerged from experience with oral contraceptives. It is not a good idea to smoke cigarettes while using estrogen—cigarettes and estrogen together may increase the likelihood of heart attack and other vascular problems. Cigarette smoking also decreases the effectiveness of ET; higher doses are needed to produce beneficial actions.

CAUTIONS

ET should be stopped when blood clots in the veins or arteries are most likely to occur; for example, when surgery or bed rest for more than several days is anticipated. Women receiving ET should avoid prolonged sitting without leg exercise, especially during air, rail, or road travel or when doing sedentary work, since the risk of clots is heightened. Becoming dehydrated also predisposes to clots in the leg veins. Walking frequently and drinking water can help prevent clotting.

There are some disadvantages to ET once it is begun; side effects can occur. If the most widely accepted way to use estrogens is followed, a woman will continue to have menstruallike bleeding—but she cannot become pregnant if she is truly menopausal—and a woman receiving estrogens must have regular medical checkups. On the other hand, one must consider the benefits of diminishing the likelihood of vertebral crush fractures and a broken hip and improving the quality of life by preventing disturbing menopausal symptoms. For this reason, *ET becomes a very personal decision that a woman must make only after she understands the benefits and side effects and is willing to adhere strictly to the advice of her physician.*

Although serious side effects of ET are very uncommon, one would not advocate estrogen to prevent bone loss in a woman who was most unlikely to develop osteoporosis. As far as the bones are concerned, estrogen is best reserved for women whose chances of developing osteoporosis are high. At high risk are women who experience an early menopause (for example, those who had an oophorectomy before age forty) and thin or petite Caucasian or Asian women, particularly if they have other high-risk traits, such as a long history of cigarette smoking. At low risk would be stout or heavy-boned black women with a menopause at the usual age. Estrogen is commonly used to prevent further bone loss in women who have osteoporosis; for example, some experts would regard a sixty-five-year-old woman with one or several crush fractures as a candidate for ET. As described in chapter 5, scientists know many of the factors that influence the chances that osteoporosis will develop, but assessment of risk is not foolproof—there are no guarantees. Each woman, under guidance from her physician, must make this highly personal and individual decision. Measurement of bone mass will aid in determining if a woman already has too little bone tissue and can be used to check on the status of her bones periodically, thereby finding out whether ET is working. Soon, urine and blood tests will be available to discover how fast a postmenopausal woman is losing bone tissue. These tests will be easily obtained in the doctor's office and relatively inexpensive and may help in diagnosing the "fast loser." "Fast losers" have more calcium in their urine and lower levels of estrogen in their blood than "slow losers."

Additional side effects of estrogen are headaches, including migraine headaches; tumors of the liver, which are very rare and usually not cancerous; nausea; vomiting; bloating; swelling of the ankles and feet; weight gain; breast soreness; brown spots on the skin; a tendency to sunburn easily; eye irritation with contact lenses; depression; and blood clots. These are most unlikely to occur with modern approaches to ET, and some will disappear when the estrogen preparation is changed or a lower dose used. Women using ET may experience abnormal vaginal bleeding—excessive bleeding or bleeding that occurs unexpectedly, for example, on days that estrogen is taken. When that happens, a physician should be contacted.

A woman should also seek medical attention for unexplained coughing; coughing up blood; pain in a calf, thigh, or groin; chest pain or heaviness; heart pounding; shortness of breath; yellow skin or eyes; severe headache; dizziness; fainting; change in vision; weakness; numbness; difficulty speaking; swelling of the legs; a lump in the breast; or breast discharge. Women must also be sure to tell their physicians *before* starting ET if they have had any of these symptoms.

ENDOMETRIAL DISORDERS

Estrogen normally stimulates the growth of endometrial tissue (the lining of the uterus) during the first phase of the menstrual cycle. During the latter phase, estrogen levels decline, and progesterone levels rise. Progesterone prepares the lining to be shed. When the lining is stimulated by estrogen alone, it thickens and does not shed properly. Sometimes, the estrogen-stimulated endometrium becomes too thick or actually develops abnormalities that can progress to cancer. Also at risk are women who are obese; have never been pregnant; or who have high blood pressure, diabetes mellitus, or gallstones. Abnormal vaginal bleeding—bleeding at the wrong time or for too long—can suggest the presence of a thickened, perhaps abnormal endometrium and makes notifying a physician mandatory. The diagnosis is made by taking a sample of the endometrial tissue (biopsy).

A woman using estrogen alone is much more likely than a nonuser to develop endometrial cancer. This kind of cancer is usually detected in its earliest stages, and most studies indicate a very high cure rate. Estrogen users need not suffer from this side effect if they also take progesterone. Studies have indicated that menopausal women who use both estrogen and progesterone are protected from endometrial cancer, perhaps because progesterone causes complete shedding of the estrogen-thickened endometrium so that cancer cannot develop. There is, of course, no guarantee. For this reason, frequent medical checkups are necessary, and some experts advocate annual biopsy of the endometrium in women receiving estrogen. The Food and Drug Administration agrees that progesterone is a useful companion to ET. Progesterone has its own side effects—including pain during menstruation, premenstrual tension, swelling, bloating, and breast tenderness—but these are uncommon, and they usually disappear when the progesterone preparation is changed or the dose adjusted. One should also know that progesterone may cancel the possible beneficial effects of estrogen on blood cholesterol levels.

Women who have had a hysterectomy incur no risk of uterine cancer (and do not need progesterone). If progesterone is later found to reduce bone loss in itself, it may be recommended to women who have had a hysterectomy who are at highest risk for osteoporosis.

BREAST CANCER

Estrogen at recommended doses has not been found to increase the overall risk of breast cancer in postmenopausal women. Comparison studies of thousands of estrogen users and nonusers point to the safety of ET in this regard. Researchers do not know whether estrogen may cause a small increase in breast cancer risk in certain women whose chances of breast cancer are already high. Despite many studies, there is still uncertainty about whether prolonged ET, more than ten years, will increase breast cancer likelihood—the possibility of a slight increase in risk cannot be eliminated. However, disturbing menopausal symptoms have usually disappeared after ten years, and reducing bone loss with estrogen for that period of time is likely to reduce the chances of osteoporosis sharply.

Since an unsuspected breast cancer may be present when estrogen therapy is started, all women contemplating ET should have a complete breast examination, including a mammogram (a detailed X-ray study of the breasts) and frequent exams thereafter. According to the American Cancer Society, all women over the age of fifty should have an annual mammogram, whether or not they are using estrogen.

ESTROGEN AND PROGESTERONE PREPARATIONS

There are many different estrogen preparations, natural and synthetic, and various ways of administering them: oral tablets, topical creams, transdermal preparations that enter the body simply when applied to the skin (now available as an adhesive patch), injectables, suppositories, and vaginal implants. The Food and Drug Administration has approved only oral, short-acting estrogen to treat osteoporosis. Some women find it more convenient to apply a skin patch several times weekly than to take a pill daily. This form of estrogen is now being tested to find out whether it will reduce bone loss, whether it has fewer side effects than oral preparations, and whether it will cause beneficial changes in blood cholesterol. There is some reason to believe that transdermal estrogens, like their orally administered counterparts, will reduce bone loss, but the effect remains unproven.

Bones are sensitive to estrogen, and a moderately low estrogen dose is all that is needed to reduce bone loss. In fact, the FDA requires that oral estrogen preparations be proven to decrease bone loss at a low dose before they can be advocated for osteoporosis. Conjugated estrogens (a group of estrogen molecules obtained from animals) have been shown to be effective against osteoporosis at a low daily dose (0.625 milligrams). Results of recent studies suggest that other estrogen preparations will be effective at a low dose as well. Higher doses may be required to eliminate disturbing menopausal symptoms. For prevention of symptoms, one should begin with a low dose and increase it if necessary. As for progesterone, several preparations (progestogens) are available to protect the endometrium.

Cycles

Estrogens are usually taken on calendar days 1 to 25, and progesterone tablets are added on calendar days 12 or 13. There is a brief rest each month during which no medication is taken and menstrual bleeding occurs. Other cycles can be used.

Continuous Therapy

Some women are relieved when menopause occurs. For them, it means the end of monthly periods. They do not look forward to bleeding again and may not accept estrogen therapy. This is particularly true if estrogen is not started soon after menopause. (Of course, such women should consider what life would be like with a hunched back or a broken hip.) Scientists are now testing a program called continuous therapy to provide ET without bleeding. This involves taking a low dose of estrogen and progesterone every day, with no cycles and therefore no time-out. Generally, there is some intermittent bleeding for three to six months, but it is then virtually eliminated. Studies indicate that women using this approach have good control of disturbing menopausal symptoms.

GENERIC ESTROGEN PREPARATIONS

Drugs manufactured and sold by various manufacturers have trade names that clearly identify them as specific products, carefully tested and marketed only after intensive examination and approval by the FDA. These specific products are protected by patents, which means that other companies cannot make them without the approval of the company that holds the patent.

When the patent on a specific drug expires, other companies may sell the product but cannot use its trade name. This new product is known as a generic, since its name is that of the general chemical compound or compounds in the drug. Often, it is sold at a lower price than the original product. To be reliable, generic preparations must have the same effects on the body as the original and be just as safe. A physician can provide information about which generic preparations have been found to be equal to the trade-named estrogens. Some have not.

CALCIUM AND EXERCISE WITH ESTROGEN THERAPY

Some members of the health care community oppose ET because of its side effects. The suggestion has been made that a high calcium intake and a vigorous exercise program will suffice to reduce postmenopausal bone loss. However, increasing intake of calcium, even to very high levels, does not appear to substitute for ET in preventing bone loss during the postmenopausal period. One study has shown that an adequate intake of calcium is needed for ET to work best, and a high intake of calcium reduces the dose of estrogen needed to diminish bone loss. Exercise may help as well. However, approaches that exclude estrogen have not yet been found to be nearly as effective as ET in the five to ten years following menopause.

12 • *Nonestrogen Prevention and Treatment— Established and Experimental*

Maintaining adequate calcium nutrition, obtaining regular weight-bearing exercise, and avoiding habits such as cigarette smoking and alcohol abuse are reasonable strategies to prevent bone loss, but their effectiveness is not guaranteed. By contrast, estrogen therapy is the most reliable way to preserve bone mass, but some women who are at risk for osteoporosis cannot or will not use estrogens, and men are not eligible. Furthermore, there is no evidence that estrogens will rebuild a skeleton already weakened by osteoporosis.

PREVENTION

These considerations have prompted a continuing scientific search for nonestrogenic agents that can diminish bone loss and for those that can stimulate new bone formation. That search has yielded one useful inhibitor of bone loss, calcitonin, and other approaches that are in the final stages of testing. Other possible bone-preserving agents under scientific study are anabolic steroids, compounds that resemble vitamin D, and certain diuretic drugs.

Calcitonin

A synthetic form of calcitonin, the hormone that blocks bone resorption, has been shown to diminish bone loss when administered to individuals in the earliest stages of osteoporosis. Studies indicate less bone loss in some persons treated with calcitonin than in untreated persons over a period of nearly three years; the decreases were of such magnitude that, if persistent, they would reduce the future likelihood of fractures. The FDA has approved calcitonin for use in treating osteoporosis. Calcitonin is quite safe. Side effects usually have been infrequent and minor: transient flushing of the face, an occasional upset stomach, a temporary sensation of numbness and tingling of the hands and feet soon after its administration, and other inconveniences.

Calcitonin treatment has several drawbacks. First, it must be given by injection, at a minimum of three times weekly. However, an intranasal (snuff) preparation, eliminating the need for injection, is now being tested. Second, currently available preparations are quite expensive, certainly beyond the financial means of some people. Third, it is not certain whether its effects will persist for longer than several years, even with continuing use. Calcitonin is an accepted treatment for another skeletal disease, Paget's disease, which is not related to osteoporosis. Although calcitonin is very effective in that condition, some patients become unresponsive to it after one or two years and "escape" from its beneficial effects. Long-term studies are now under way to discover whether persons with osteoporosis will experience a like reaction. Fourth, some people just don't experience the protective effect of calcitonin in the first place—so-called nonresponders. Recent studies show that individuals who have a rapid rate of bone remodeling (see pages 20–22) respond more favorably to calcitonin.

Eligible for calcitonin therapy are men and women at high risk for osteoporosis—or persons who already have osteoporosis, in whom it is used to prevent further bone loss. Calcitonin is not likely to help in advanced osteoporosis, when bone loss has been severe. The possibility that it can promote bone formation and actually increase bone mass is being tested. Calcitonin sometimes has an additional effect that makes it useful in osteoporosis—pain relief. Consequently, some patients with osteoporosis have found that calcitonin reduces back pain suffered after a crush fracture. Calcitonin may emerge as a bone loss preventive in patients who are immobilized or who are being treated with bone-wasting cortisonelike drugs for various medical illnesses. One recent study suggests that estrogen and calcitonin may be more effective in reducing postmenopausal bone loss than estrogen alone.

Anabolic Steroids

Anabolic steroids, patterned after the male hormone testosterone, are familiar to many as the drugs used by weight lifters and certain athletes to aid in building muscle tissue. They are prescribed by gynecologists to treat endometriosis. Evidence indicates that these agents decrease bone loss in postmenopausal women and may actually cause new bone to form. The FDA has not approved their use for osteoporosis in the United States—in part because of potentially serious side effects. These same side effects argue against their use as bodybuilding aids but have not curtailed illicit sales for that purpose. Women exposed to anabolic steroids may experience a mild degree of masculinization—principally growth of hair on the face—and some of these agents can cause a higher level of blood cholesterol than women generally have.

1,25 Vitamin D

Two relatives of vitamin D have been tested as treatments for osteoporosis—1,25 dihydroxy vitamin D (the active form of vitamin D manufactured in the kidney) and 1 alpha hydroxy vitamin D (a synthetic version of "1,25"). Neither compound is recommended nor approved for use, since effectiveness has not been proven and since calcium may build up in the urine (causing kidney stones) and blood too easily in treated individuals.

Thiazides

Diuretic drugs, often used to treat high blood pressure, also influence the kidneys' metabolism of calcium. One class of diuretics, the thiazides, actually reduces calcium elimination by the kidneys, and the conservation of calcium has been thought to inhibit bone loss. Test results in osteoporosis, however, have conflicted—some studies showing reduced bone loss, others showing no effect. Until this discrepancy is resolved through further research, thiazides should not be used to prevent osteoporosis.

TREATMENT

If the number of agents known to prevent osteoporosis is small, even shorter is the list of approaches to rebuilding bone. Three strategies are now being investigated: pulse therapy with diphosphonates and ADFR, fluoride therapy, and parathyroid hormone therapy. Anabolic steroids (see above) may also be bone-building agents.

Pulse Therapy

Diphosphonates, a class of drugs, are chemical compounds that are potent inhibitors of bone resorption. Like calcitonin, they are effective treatments for patients with Paget's disease. Etidronate is the diphosphonate that the FDA has approved for treating Paget's disease. Diphosphonates are active when taken by mouth, and side effects have been infrequent and minor. Recently, diphosphonates have been tested for their ability to block bone loss and actually build new bone tissue in patients with osteoporosis. To accomplish this, scientists conceived of a novel approach called pulse, or intermittent, therapy and a complex variant of pulse therapy termed ADFR. In pulse therapy, a diphosphonate is administered sporadically, for example, daily for two consecutive weeks out of every two months. The theory underlying this strategy is that the blocking of bone resorption at all remodeling "factories" after it has begun but before it is finished will have triggered the same amount of bone formation, or repair, as would have occurred if resorption were complete. Thus, more bone is made than was taken away. Cycles of pulse therapy are repeated every two to three months, producing small, stepwise increases in the amount of bone tissue. After two to three years, one might be able to see substantial increases.

ADFR is a modified version of pulse therapy, in which the remodeling "factories" are turned on, or *A*ctivated, before the diphosphonate is given to inhibit, or *D*epress, bone resorption. Then, no treatment is given—bones are *F*ree of therapy so that bone formation can occur—and finally, the cycle is *R*epeated every two to three months (*A*ctivate, *D*epress, *F*ree, and *R*epeat). Calcitonin or other agents could be used in place of diphosphonates to depress bone resorption. But the diphosphonates are being widely studied, with promising but *very preliminary* results.

Fluoride Therapy

Fluoride is an element that has a strong affinity for calcium-containing tissues, particularly tooth enamel and bone. Many communities add fluoride to the drinking water because it hardens dental enamel and reduces cavity formation. Fluoride-containing toothpastes serve the same purpose. These amounts of fluoride (one part fluoride per million parts drinking water) have not been proven to affect the skeleton. But ingestion of greater amounts of fluoride is known to stimulate bone formation—actually to promote the accumulation of new bone tissue.

The first clues to this effect came from studies of people who were exposed to extraordinarily large fluoride doses—usually by drinking fluoride-contaminated well water (containing ten or more parts per million of fluoride). An excessive amount of abnormal bone tissue accumulated in people so exposed. Overgrowth of the vertebrae caused severe pressure on the spinal cord and nerves resulting in permanent numbness and paralysis. In searching for a cure for osteoporosis, scientists reasoned that administration of fluoride in moderate doses to persons with osteoporosis might make bone stronger but not abnormal. These scientists took great care to provide the fluoride-treated persons with sufficient calcium so that maximum bone hardness could be achieved. The results of these initial studies have been promising. Fluoride, given as sodium fluoride at doses of 50–80 milligrams a day in association with adequate calcium nutrition (1,000 or more milligrams of calcium daily) increases the amount of bone tissue in the vertebrae of most, but not all, subjects.

Fluoride treatment of osteoporosis is still experimental, however, for it has not been proven to prevent osteoporosis-related fractures. Furthermore, serious side effects are common, such as stomach ailments and pain in the feet and knees caused by small fractures in these weight-bearing bones. New, more slowly absorbed preparations do not appear to irritate the stomach. It is possible that fluoride builds trabecular bone (as in the spine) but not cortical bone (as in the bones of the hips, legs, and feet). Some persons just don't respond to fluoride at all, for reasons that are not understood. Fortunately, two large-scale studies on fluoride in the treatment of osteoporosis are now being conducted with the support of the National Institutes of Health, and the results will be available in about two years.

Parathyroid Hormone Therapy

Parathyroid hormone is the main stimulator of bone resorption in the body, and when overproduced in patients with hyperparathyroidism, it causes bone loss. These are scientific facts. Nevertheless, scientists know that injection of low doses of a synthetic parathyroid hormone preparation actually boosts bone formation. As with fluoride use, it is too soon to tell whether parathyroid hormone will work safely and whether it will be an inexpensive option for individuals with osteoporosis.

There are, then, alternatives to ET for the woman who is a candidate for osteoporosis. Other agents that can reduce bone loss are available or in the final stages of study. Safe drug treatments to rebuild the skeleton are not yet available. But there is still hope for individuals who already have severe bone loss—one can learn to live with osteoporosis.

13 • Living with Osteoporosis—How to Prevent Fractures

Injuries due to falling are a major problem in an aging population. About one-fifth of older persons who live independently fall each year, and injuries from falls are significant causes of suffering and even death among individuals over sixty-five. Evidence indicates that falls increase in frequency and severity with advancing age. Falls trigger most of the nearly 250,000 hip fractures sustained annually by individuals with osteoporosis in the United States, as well as countless injuries of other types. Older individuals who fall repeatedly or sustain serious injury can become afraid to walk. Literally immobilized by fear, their quality of life deteriorates.

Falls and the injuries they cause can be prevented. Readers who are over sixty-five should understand why they are more likely to fall than young adults and how to prevent falls. Younger readers are urged to convey this information to their older relatives and close friends.

Three factors increase the tendency to fall with advancing age. *First*, reflexes and muscle strength that help maintain equilibrium diminish in old age. *Second*, older persons are more likely to have disorders that disturb balance. *Third*, older individuals commonly take drugs that cause dizziness or that blunt equilibrium reflexes. Environmental factors may interact with the foregoing circumstances to increase even further the likelihood of falling. In addition, loss of fat and muscle tissue with advancing age removes "protective padding," increasing the chances of injury during a fall.

REFLEXES AND MUSCLE STRENGTH

Coordinated actions of the nervous and cardiovascular systems are responsible for maintaining balance. The eyes, as well as internal position-cuing organs, and blood pressure sensors instantly detect any rapid change in position, triggering reflexes to induce the muscular activity that restores balance. Good muscle tone allows these reflexes to work effectively. Natural slowing of these mechanisms and loss of muscle tissue with advancing age need not jeopardize one's safety, since much can be done to reduce the likelihood of falling. Obtaining the proper diagnosis and correction of visual disturbances; exercising regularly to maintain good muscle tone, flexible joints, and blood pressure reflexes; and even something as trivial as the frequent removal of earwax can protect against falling.

Falls are most likely to occur upon arising after sleep or after a meal. Lowering of blood pressure appears to be responsible for the dizziness that occurs at those times in some otherwise healthy older individuals. Drinking a cup of caffeinated coffee has been suggested but not proven to help prevent dizziness after eating.

DISORDERS THAT DISTURB BALANCE

Potentially treatable disorders of the heart, nervous system, thyroid, and metabolic system (diabetes mellitus) are among the conditions that can impair balance reflexes. The warning signs of balance disorders are blurring of vision, blind spots, light-headedness, dizziness, palpitations, skipped heartbeats, weakness, numbness, difficulty in walking, and shakiness.

DRUGS

Older people take more drugs and are more likely to take balance-disturbing drugs than younger people. Many kinds of drugs can cause dizziness or light-headedness: sleeping medications, mood elevators, tranquilizers, muscle relaxants, diuretics, and drugs used to treat high blood pressure. Moreover, certain combinations of drugs can further increase the risk of falling. Needed medications should not be avoided, but only the safest possible regimen should be used. *Under no circumstances should a recommended drug be stopped without a doctor's advice.* Dizziness, light-headedness, weakness, or any disturbance in equilibrium—and experiencing falling, of course—must prompt a thorough medical evaluation. Any such problems should be reported to a physician without delay.

ALCOHOL

In addition to prescribed and over-the-counter drugs, *alcoholic beverages, when used in excess, are particularly dangerous for older people.* Alcohol can further disturb the already impaired balance of the older person. Furthermore, the initial "high" and the subsequent depression, disorientation, and fatigue may prevent the exercising of caution in action and decision making. One is more likely to take chances and less likely to recognize hazards. Since alcohol is a depressant, it is particularly dangerous when taken with other depressants, such as sleeping medications and tranquilizers. The chances of falling are much greater under these circumstances. (It is the view of the authors of this book that there is no "safe" amount of alcohol that can be used with other drugs.)

COLD TEMPERATURES

Prolonged exposure to cold temperatures in the environment can disturb balance. Elderly people cannot tolerate the cold as well as younger people. Their body temperatures actually fall, a condition known as hypothermia. Hypothermia can produce dizziness and falling (and, ultimately, loss of consciousness and death). Individuals are particularly susceptible to accidental hypothermia during sleep and when they have consumed an excessive amount of alcohol, which causes the body to lose heat. Dysfunction of home heating systems or failure to use the system properly can be responsible for such exposure. It is particularly important that the temperature in the bedroom not be lower than sixty-five degrees Fahrenheit during sleep. Individuals whose limited budget may deprive them of adequate heating should contact their Area Agency on Aging for advice.

HOME HAZARDS

"Most accidents happen in the home" is an old but true adage. A large proportion of the falls and hip fractures that occur among the elderly take place in the home. Many of these falls and fractures result from encounters with hazardous conditions in the home that have not been recognized and remedied. People spend much time at home. In comfortable and familiar surroundings, hazards are invisible. Enjoying a safe home environment requires an awareness of dangerous conditions and their correction, if possible.

Four main home hazards are inadequate lighting, absence of sturdy support and climbing aids, slippery floor surfaces, and obstacles to safe walking.

Lighting

Homes should be equipped with adequate lighting both outside and inside, particularly in stairways and hallways. Poor lighting is almost as bad as none at all, since it casts confusing shadows. Strong but low-glare bulbs are most helpful. Inexpensive night-lights can be installed in every room to illuminate places where bright lights are not needed. Placement of light switches is very important for safety. Switches should be in easy-to-reach places at entrances to all rooms and to the garage, at the top *and* bottom of each stairway, and within easy reach of the bed. A workable flashlight should be kept at locations where lighting is inadequate. Painting steps and risers contrasting bright colors can amplify the beneficial effect of lighting.

Support and Climbing Aids

Support aids are needed for safety. Indoor and outdoor steps should have sturdy handrails from top to bottom. Handrails should be in good repair, firmly fixed to the wall or support; should extend along the entire length of the stairs; and, most important, should be used. It may seem quicker to carry all those bundles in one trip, but it is much safer to carry only as much as you can and still grip one of the stair railings. Bathtubs, shower walls, and the walls next to the bathtub should be equipped with easily reached handgrips and toilets with sturdy side arms. A waterproof stool or small chair in the shower is also helpful. Anyone with any difficulty arising or walking should consider using a lightweight aluminum walker or, as is more acceptable, a cane that has a no-slip tip. The advice of a health professional should be sought if a walking aid is desirable.

Use of chairs or other inadequate climbing aids is an invitation to falling. A sturdy, low step stool with handrails is the safest climbing aid. An even more sensible idea is to store things where they can be reached without climbing.

Slippery Floor Surfaces

Slippery floors are particularly dangerous. Bathroom, kitchen, and basement floors should be kept dry. Bathtubs and showers should have nonslip surfaces. Smooth tile floors should be made as safe as possible with nonskid rugs or mats. Hard floors can be treacherous, especially when highly polished. There are preparations other than wax (such as chemical sealants) that make the floor look good and are not as dangerous.

Obstacles to Safe Walking

Rugs or mats that slip easily should be eliminated or stabilized with a nonslip pad. A new rubber webbing is now on the market for this purpose; it is thin and doesn't raise the height of the rug. Shag rugs and damaged or torn rugs are also hazardous, especially on stairs; projecting nails and raised carpet edges are likewise treacherous. Stairs should not be covered with deep pile carpeting or patterned or dark-colored carpeting, which can cause a person to misjudge steps. Outdoor steps should be painted with white or light-colored paint that does not produce a slick surface when dry and should have adhesive strips affixed to them. Sand may be mixed with paint to reduce slipperiness.

Additional home hazards for both young and old include appliance cords, especially long extension and phone cords, low-lying furniture, children's toys, four-legged pets, and protruding shelves and cupboards, decorative hangings, or other overhanging items. Sticky drawers or doors that yield suddenly when pulled can precipitate a fall.

IMPROPER CLOTHING

Improper clothing can jeopardize safety. Shoes with high heels or with little support should be avoided. Shoes with low heels and sure-grip soles allow the safest possible movement, and those shoes should be used; walking in stockinged feet is dangerous. Pants that are too long or have a loose cuff can catch a heel. Tight-fitting jackets restrict arm movement. A little-known clothing hazard is a tight girdle, which can cause dizziness by restricting respiration. A good rule of thumb is, If it isn't comfortable, it probably isn't safe.

STRESSES ON THE SPINE

Crush fractures of the spine are more difficult to prevent than other fractures. They often occur during common activities that place several stresses on the spine—for example, lifting, twisting, straining to get out of bed, arising from a chair, or sitting down abruptly, particularly on a hard surface. Individuals with osteoporosis are advised to rise and sit carefully and avoid lifting heavy objects.

AIDS TO SUMMON HELP

In the event of a fall or other accident in the home, some individuals, particularly those who live alone, may not be physically able to get help. To prevent this situation, older people may want to consider subscribing to a telephone monitoring service, which will make daily or more frequent telephone calls to the home to make sure that all is well; if there is no answer, emergency personnel will be notified. Also available are devices worn on the body that can summon help at the touch of a finger. To find out more about these kinds of aids (and to get answers to additional questions about home safety), contact the Area Agency on Aging.

It is possible to be protected without fear of activity. In fact, regular exercise that maintains muscle tone and strength, undertaken only with a doctor's advice, helps prevent falling and injury. Inactivity can be more dangerous.

A PERSONAL HAZARD CHECKLIST

- ☐ You have had a recent medical checkup, including an eye examination.
- ☐ You are following your doctor's safety suggestions about balance-disturbing medical problems and drugs.
- ☐ You are not drinking alcoholic beverages in excess.
- ☐ You are not wearing dangerous clothing or shoes.
- ☐ Your vision and hearing have been checked recently and are corrected appropriately.
- ☐ You are wearing your glasses as prescribed.
- ☐ You are very cautious when rising, standing, and walking after meals and after lying down or sleeping.
- ☐ You are using safe walking aids as recommended by a health professional.

A HOME HAZARD CHECKLIST

Lighting

☐ Dwelling well lit inside and out
☐ Adequate stairway lighting
☐ Light switches easy to reach and appropriately placed
    ☐ top and bottom of staircase
    ☐ entrance to rooms and garage
    ☐ near each bed

Support and Climbing Aids

☐ Sturdy handrails on all stairs
☐ Handgrips next to tub and shower, and side arms on toilet
☐ Walker or cane(s) with no-slip tip available if needed
☐ Sturdy, low step stool with handrails

Slippery Surfaces

☐ Nonslip bathroom, kitchen, basement, bathtub, and shower floors
☐ Water leaks repaired
☐ Dwelling well heated
☐ Carpeting not shag, deep pile, patterned, or dark-colored and in good repair
☐ Floor tile or wood not highly polished or waxed
☐ Slippery floors covered with nonskid mats
☐ Outdoor steps nonslip and painted a light color

Other Hazards

☐ Appliance cords (long extension lines and phone cords) eliminated or not exposed
☐ Low-lying furniture, protruding shelves, cupboards, or wall hangings away from traffic zones
☐ Drawers and doors not sticky
☐ Pets and toys not underfoot

14 • New Thrusts in Current Research

Osteoporosis has attracted considerable attention in the past few years. One of the benefits of that attention has been a vigorous search for new understanding about the disorder—and for new methods of predicting risk, of prevention, and of treatment. Medical research has yielded considerable new knowledge in these areas. But there is much more to learn. Consider what is needed: (1) an accurate, reliable, inexpensive way to determine a person's risk for developing osteoporosis and to measure the amount of bone tissue the person has, and (2) effective, safe, inexpensive strategies to maximize bone strength during the formative years, to prevent bone loss, and to restore lost bone tissue.

Scientists, trained and supported principally by funds from the federal government—and to a smaller degree by private industry and nonprivate agencies, mainly the National Osteoporosis Foundation (NOF)—are attacking these problems from three standpoints: (1) bone research, conducting fundamental studies to learn more about the nature of bone tissue and how it grows and is remodeled; (2) technical research, developing new technologies to measure bone tissue; and (3) clinical research, studying risk and protective factors and testing agents for and approaches to modifying the amount and strength of bone tissue. Very promising new leads have appeared in each area.

BONE RESEARCH

Recently, researchers have learned that bone remodeling is under the control of chemicals produced by bone cells themselves, including proteins called growth factors and special fatty substances called prostaglandins. Some growth factor proteins are actually stored in bone tissue. It is theorized that they are released from storage when a bone is broken, whereupon they encourage the healing process, the creation of new bone. Physical exercise, which puts pressure on bone cells, may be another way of stimulating the release of growth-promoting chemicals. The job of researchers is to harvest these growth proteins in pure form, to learn how they act, and to see whether doctors can use them to reduce the losses of bone associated with aging and thereby "heal" or "cure" osteoporosis.

Another task is to understand the ways in which physical exercise affects bone. Recent discoveries indicate that stretching bone tissue creates tiny electrical signals, not unlike static electricity, which in turn stimulate the release of growth-stimulating chemicals. Orthopedic surgeons now use electrical currents to hasten the healing of fractures that are mending too slowly. Once understood, the electrical and chemical processes involved in bone growth can be harnessed to prevent and treat osteoporosis.

TECHNICAL RESEARCH

Novel methods of measuring bone mass and monitoring the rate of bone loss are being sought. Improved technology may reduce the cost of testing while enhancing accuracy so that these tests can be applied to individuals who do not have the recognized risk factors—that is, evaluation of medical history, family history, and current state of health does not place them at high risk. This clinical assessment is far from accurate; some individuals who appear to be at low risk may nevertheless have osteoporosis or may be losing bone rapidly, but existing methods for bone mass measurement are simply too expensive to use to test everyone. Cheaper, accurate approaches that will make widespread testing more reasonable are on the horizon. At the same time, investigators are developing several new chemical tests that can indicate how fast a patient is losing bone tissue. For example, available in the near future will be blood and urine tests that disclose which postmenopausal women are losing bone fast, thus making them likely candidates for osteoporosis and therefore for estrogen and/or calcitonin therapy or other preventive strategies.

CLINICAL RESEARCH

To discover who is at greatest risk, long before osteoporosis is established, is a crucial goal of modern research. Scientists hope that the new measuring and monitoring methods will enable medical professionals to learn more about who is and who is not at risk and why.

Attention also is being paid to another key aspect of risk—the risk for fracture. Not all individuals with osteoporosis will actually suffer a broken bone—in fact, fractures will occur in only a minority. Knowing who is most likely to fracture becomes very important. Since a fall is the cause of virtually all broken wrists and most broken hips, researchers have undertaken studies to learn about the causes of falls and what can be done to prevent falling. The recognition that some older individuals may be likely to fall after eating because of a drop in blood pressure represents the kind of information that may aid in preventing many serious injuries.

The exact cause of osteoporosis is not known. It would be much easier for doctors to develop more effective, safer ways of preventing and treating osteoporosis if they understood why everyone loses bone with advancing age, why bone is lost so rapidly after the menopause, and why estrogens reduce that bone loss. An important breakthrough, the culmination of many years of research, has been the recent evidence that estrogens may influence bone tissue directly. Bone cells appear to contain molecules, called receptors, that recognize and attach to estrogen, much like a lock and key. It may now be possible to tailor new chemicals that will fit into the estrogen receptor and will diminish bone loss, like estrogen, but have no side effects.

Research is also being done in the area of "protective factors" other than estrogen. Scientists are endeavoring to understand how calcium affects bone tissue and why obese individuals and blacks are less likely than thin, Caucasian, and Asian people to develop osteoporosis.

The challenge to the scientific and medical community is to eliminate osteoporosis. These and other lines of inquiry in current research offer great promise toward that goal in our lifetime.

Readers who wish to keep up with new developments in research on osteoporosis may contact the National Osteoporosis Foundation, 1625 Eye Street, N.W., Suite 1011, Washington, DC 20006.

Bibliography

Avioli, L. V. *Calcium and osteoporosis.* 1984. *Annual Review of Nutrition* 4:471-491.

Consensus Development Conference on Osteoporosis. 1984. *Journal of the American Medical Association* 252:799-802.

Current Perspectives in the Management of the Menopausal and Postmenopausal Patient—Symposium. 1987. *American Journal of Obstetrics and Gynecology* 156:1279-1356.

Ettinger, B.; Genant, H. K.; and Cann, C. E. 1985. Long-term estrogen replacement therapy prevents bone loss and fractures. *Annals of Internal Medicine* 102:319-324.

———. 1987. Postmenopausal bone loss is prevented by treatment with low-dosage estrogen with calcium. *Annals of Internal Medicine* 106:40-45.

Gruber, H. E.; Ivey, J. L.; and Baylink, D. J. 1984. Long-term calcitonin therapy in postmenopausal osteoporosis. *Metabolism* 33:295-303.

Heaney, R. P. Calcium, bone health, and osteoporosis. In *Bone and Mineral Research* 4, W. A. Peck, ed., 255-301. Amsterdam: Elsevier Science Publishers, 1986.

Heaney, R. P.; Recker, R. R.; and Saville, P. D. 1978. Menopausal changes in calcium balance performance. *Journal of Laboratory and Clinical Medicine* 92:953-963.

Johnston, C. C., Jr. Studies on prevention of age-related bone loss. In *Bone and Mineral Research* 3, W. A. Peck, ed., 233-257. Amsterdam: Elsevier Science Publishers, 1985.

Kaufman, D. W.; Miller, D. R.; Rosenberg, L.; Helmrich, S. P.; Stolley, P.; Schottenfeld, D.; and Shapiro, S. 1984. Noncontraceptive estrogen use and the risk of breast cancer. *Journal of the American Medical Association* 252:63–67.

Kiel, D. P.; Felson, D. T.; Anderson, J. J.; Wilson, P. W. F.; and Moskowitz, M. A. 1987. Hip fracture and the use of estrogens in postmenopausal women: the Framingham study. *New England Journal of Medicine* 317:1169–1174.

Matkovic, V.; Kostial, K.; Simonivoc, I.; Buzina, R.; Brodarec, A.; and Nordin, B. E. C. 1979. Bone status and fracture rates in two regions of Yugoslavia. *American Journal of Clinical Nutrition* 32:540–549.

Mazess, R. B. The noninvasive measurement of skeletal mass. In *Bone and Mineral Research Annual* 1, W. A. Peck, ed., 223–279. Amsterdam: Excerpta Medica, 1983.

Peck, W. A.; Riggs, B. L.; and Bell, N. H. *Physician's Resource Manual on Osteoporosis; a Decision-Making Guide.* Washington, D.C.: National Osteoporosis Foundation, 1987.

Pocock, N. A.; Eisman, J. A.; Yeates, M. G.; Sambrook, P. N.; and Eberi, S. 1986. Physical fitness is a major determinant of femoral neck and lumbar spine bone mineral density. *Journal of Clinical Investigation* 78:618–621.

Riggs, B. L. Treatment of osteoporosis with sodium fluoride: an appraisal. In *Bone and Mineral Research* 2, W. A. Peck, ed., 366–393. Amsterdam: Elsevier Science Publishers, 1984.

Riis, B.; Thomsen, K.; and Christiansen, C. 1987. Does calcium supplementation prevent postmenopausal bone loss? A double-blind controlled study. *New England Journal of Medicine* 316:173–177.

U.S. Department of Health and Human Services, National Institute of Arthritis, Musculoskeletal and Skin Diseases. *Osteoporosis; Cause, Treatment, Prevention.* Washington, D.C., 1986. NIH Publication No. 86-2226.

Weinstein, M. C., and Schiff, I. 1983. Cost-effectiveness of hormone therapy in the menopause. *Obstetrical and Gynecological Survey* 38:445–455.

• Index

Accidents, home hazards, 118–20
Aerobic exercise, 88–89
Age, as risk factor for osteoporosis, 3, 32, 33
Aged, calcium consumption by, 61, 64
Alcohol
  abuse, 3, 38
  and calcium intake, 64
  effect on balance, 117
Anabolic steroids, 111
Arthritis, rheumatoid, 46–47
Atherosclerosis, 30

Balance disorders, 116–18
Biopsy, 57
Blacks, osteoporosis in, 33
Blood pressure. See also Hypertension
  effect of estrogen therapy on, 102
Bone marrow, 11
Bone mass, measurement of, 4, 53–58
Bone research, 124
Bones
  calcium content of, 23
  cells, 20
  chemical structure of, 8
  crystal, 8
  and exercise, 87–88
  as living tissue, 1–2
  loss, 56
    estrogen therapy for, 3–4
    prevention of, 5–6, 100–101
    research on, 124–25
  remodeling, 20–21, 28

Boron, 75–76
Brain, calcium requirement of, 2
Breads, calcium content of, 69
Breast cancer, 105–106
Brittle bone disease, 48

Calcitonin, 4, 24–25, 109–110
Calcium
  bone content of, 23
  deficiency, 23–24, 36–37
  dietary inadequacy of, 1–2
  diets for, 70–73
  drug effects, 64–65
  and estrogen therapy, 108
  food content, 65–74
  and food habits, 62–65
  importance of, 23–24
  levels of, 2, 59–61
  maximum intake of, 79
  side effects of, 76–79
  supplements, 5, 82–85
  and vitamin D, 80
Cancer, 77
  beneficial effect of calcium suggested, 81
  breast, 105–106
CAT scans, 55–57
Cereals
  calcium content of, 67
  sodium content of, 74
Cheeses, calcium content of, 68
Cholesterol, 99
Cigarettes
  effect on menopause, 39
  as risk factor for osteoporosis, 3, 38–39

129

Climacteric. See Menopause
Clothing, unsafe, 120
Cold, effect on balance, 117
Collagen, 8
Computed axial tomography (CAT), 55–57
Constipation, 85
Contraceptives, oral, 41
Cortisone, effect on osteoporosis, 39–40
Cushing's syndrome, 40

Dairy products, calcium content of, 68
Dehydration, 95
Diabetes, 95
Diet, as risk factor for osteoporosis, 3
Diets, 70–73
Diphosphonates, 112–13
Discs, slipped, 11
Diseases, and calcium intake, 63–64
Drugs
  effect on balance, 116–17
  effect on calcium needs, 64–65
  effect on osteoporosis, 39–40
Dual photon absorptiometry (DPA), 54

Emphysema, 48
Endometrial disorder, 104–105
Endometrium, cancer of, 6
Estrogen, 27–28, 29, 34
Estrogen exposure, 41–42
Estrogen therapy, 5, 96–108
  and calcium, 108
  and cancer of the endometrium, 6
  effect on bone loss, 3–4
  and exercise, 108
  as protective factor, 42
  side effects of, 6, 102–104
Exercise, 90–93
  benefits of, 6, 31
  and bone accumulation, 87–88, 124
  dehydration risk, 95
  and diabetics, 95
  effect on bone, 124
  and estrogen therapy, 108
  lack of, 38
  pulse rate in, 89
  as risk factor for osteoporosis, 3
  walking, 94–95

Fluoride, 113–14
Food habits, and calcium intake, 62–65
Foods, calcium content of, 65–74
Fractures, 12, 32
  hip, 17–19
  prognosis of, 3, 18
  spinal, 13, 15–17
  statistics on, 19, 115
Fruits, calcium content of, 67

Gallbladder disease, 101
Genetics, as risk factor for osteoporosis, 33
Grave's disease, 43
Growth hormone, 27

Haversian systems, 11
Heart, calcium requirement of, 2
Heredity, as risk factor for osteoporosis, 3
High blood pressure. See Hypertension
Hip fractures, 17–19
Home hazards (for accidents), 118–20

Hormones, 24–28
  as risk factor for osteoporosis, 34–36
Hydroxyapatite, 8
Hyperparathyroidism, 39
Hypertension, and calcium intake, 81
Hyperthyroidism, 39
Hysterectomy, 30

Intestinal diseases, 39, 45–46
Isometric exercise, 88

Joints, 12

Kidney disease, 48
Kidneys, calcium requirement of, 2
Kidney stones, 26, 77

Lactose intolerance, 37
Lifestyle, 37–38
Liver disease, 48

Magnesium, 79
Malabsorption, 45
Meat, calcium content of, 67, 68
Men, rate of bone loss in, 56
Menopause, 29–30, 34
  bone loss in, 97–98
  and cigarette smoking, 39
  effect on osteoporosis, 6
  false, 34–35
  heart disease, 98–99
  post, and calcium intake, 75
Menstrual cycle, 28–29
Menus, 70–73
Milk, calcium content of, 66
Minerals, 79
Muscularity, 41–42

Neuron activation, 57

Obesity, 41
Oophorectomy, 30
Oral contraceptives, 41
Oriental foods, calcium content of, 74
Osteoarthritis, 12
Osteogenesis imperfecta, 48
Osteomalacia, 39, 48–49
Osteoporosis
  age as risk factor for, 32
  in blacks, 33
  and calcium deficiency, 36–37
  and cancer, 47
  cigarette smoking as risk factor for, 3, 38–39
  and cortisone treatments, 39–40
  diagnosis, 53–58
  and estrogen exposure, 41–42
  frequency of, 3
  genetics as risk factor for, 33
  hormones as risk factor for, 34–36
  and hyperparathyroidism, 44–45
  and hyperthyroidism, 43–44
  and intestinal diseases, 45–46
  and lactose intolerance, 37
  lifestyle risk factors, 37–39
  and muscularity, 41
  and obesity, 41
  and pregnancy, 42
  prevention of, 5–6, 31
  race as risk factor for, 33
  research, 7
  and rheumatoid arthritis, 46–47
  sex as risk factor for, 33

Osteoporosis (*continued*)
  statistics, 7
  and steroid treatments, 39–40
Ovaries, 28

Parathyroid hormone, 24–25, 114
Pregnancy, 42
Progesterone, 27–28, 107
Prolactinoma, 36
Pulse rate, in exercise, 89
Pulse therapy, 112–13

Race, as risk factor for osteoporosis, 3, 33
Recommended Dietary Allowance (RDA), 59–61
Remodeling, of bones, 20–21
Rheumatoid arthritis, 46–47
Risk factors, 3–4
  age, 32
  cigarette smoking, 3, 38–39
  genetics, 33
  hormones, 34–36
  lifestyles, 37–39
  race, 33
  sex, 3, 33

Sex, as risk factor for osteoporosis, 3, 33
Sex hormones, 27–28
Single photon absorptiometry (SPA), 53–54
Skeleton, 9–12
Slipped discs, 11
Smoking
  and calcium intake, 63
  effect on menopause, 39
  as risk factor for osteoporosis, 3, 38–39
Sodium, in cereals, 74
Spine
  deformities of, 16–17
  fractures of, 13, 15–17
  stresses on, 120
Sprue, 46
Steroids, 111
  effect on osteoporosis, 39–40

Telephone monitoring services, 121
Temperature, cold
  effect on balance, 117
Testosterone, 30, 34
Thiazides, 111
Thyroid hormone, 26–27

United States Recommended Daily Allowance (USRDA), 60

Vegetables, calcium content of, 67
Vertebrae, 15–17
Vitamin D, 24–26, 111
  and calcium, 80
  excess amounts of, 80

Walking, 94–95
Women
  calcium consumption by, 61
  frequency of spinal fractures in, 13
  osteoporosis prevalence in, 2, 34
  rate of bone loss in, 56

X rays, 52

Zinc, 79, 85

About the Authors

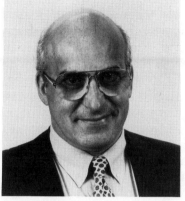
William A. Peck

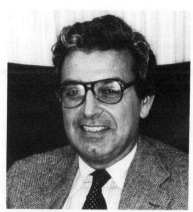
Louis V. Avioli

William A. Peck, M.D., is a physician, educator, and research scientist. He is physician-in-chief at the Jewish Hospital of Saint Louis, and the John E. and Adeline Simon professor of medicine and cochairman of the department of medicine of the Washington University School of Medicine. First president of the National Osteoporosis Foundation, Dr. Peck has discussed osteoporosis on numerous local and national TV and radio programs and has been quoted or mentioned in newspaper and magazine articles on the subject nationwide. As research scientist, he recently received a five-million-dollar grant from the National Institute on Aging to fund a five-year study on the causes and prevention of hip fractures in the elderly. Dr. Peck leads a multidisciplinary team of physicians and scientists from Jewish Hospital, the Washington University School of Medicine, and Columbia University in New York.

He has authored or coauthored more than a hundred printed selections including articles in scientific journals, book chapters, editorials, and abstracts and serves on the editorial boards of numerous scientific organizations. He has participated in and chaired many national and international scientific committees and conferences and is past president of the American Society for Bone and Mineral Research.

Having received his undergraduate degree from Harvard in 1955, Dr. Peck then graduated with honors from the University of Rochester School of Medicine and Dentistry in 1960. Among his many awards, Dr. Peck was named clinical teacher of the year by the medical students of Washington University several years ago. He lives in Town and Country, Missouri, with his wife, Patricia, who is an editor.

Louis V. Avioli, M.D., a specialist in metabolic bone disease and endocrinology, has vigorously emphasized research in his field throughout his twenty-eight-year career as a scientist, educator, and clinician. Educated at Princeton University as an undergraduate, he was named professor of medicine at Washington University School of Medicine thirteen years after his graduation from Yale Medical School in 1957. In 1975, he was named director of the then newly created Division of Bone and Mineral Metabolism at Washington University School of Medicine and the Jewish Hospital of St. Louis.

Dr. Avioli's career has spanned the international scientific community. On two occasions he accepted an invitation from the Chinese Ministry of Health to visit that country and teach its medical community about endocrinology and metabolic bone disease. He has been visiting professor to medical schools in Italy, Venezuela, South Africa, Australia, Taiwan, Japan, and Spain, and he has served as a consultant for the Medical Research Council of Canada.

Nationally, he founded and served as the first president of the American Society of Bone and Mineral Research, and he served as a member and chairman of the National Institutes of Health General Medicine Section. As a member of the National Research Council of the Space Sciences Board of the National Academy of Sciences, he has been continually involved in this country's space program. In 1983, Dr. Avioli was named one of the 120 best doctors in America by a survey of more than 400 department chairpersons and clinical program chiefs at 87 U.S. medical schools. He is the author of more than 180 original papers and of 83 chapters in various books, and he is the editor of 14 books on endocrinology or bone disease. He lives in Saint Louis, Missouri, with his wife, Joan, and has five children.

Scott, Foresman and the American Association of Retired Persons have joined together to bring you AARP Books.

 These comprehensive guides, written by experts, will help you manage your money, choose where to live, plan your estate, guard your health, and help those you care about live a better life.

835. **Osteoporosis:** *The Silent Thief. $9.95 / AARP member price $6.95.*
831. **AARP Pharmacy Service Prescription Drug Handbook.** *$13.95 / AARP member price $9.95.*
805. **The Essential Guide to Wills, Estates, Trusts and Death Taxes.** *$12.95 / AARP member price $9.45.*
834. **Homesharing and Other Lifestyle Options.** *$12.95 / AARP member price $9.45.*
808. **Survival Handbook for Widows** (and for relatives and friends who want to understand). *$5.95 / AARP member price $4.35.*
810. **Alone - Not Lonely:** *Independent Living for Women Over Fifty. $6.95 / AARP member price $4.95.*
811. **Travel Easy:** *The Practical Guide for People Over 50. $8.95 / AARP member price $6.50.*
813. **Medical and Health Guide for People Over Fifty.** *$14.95 / AARP member price $10.85.*
815. **Cataracts:** *The Complete Guide From Diagnosis to Recovery for Patients and Families. $7.95 / AARP member price $5.80.*
823. **The Inside Tract:** *Understanding and Preventing Digestive Disorders. $9.95 / AARP member price $6.95.*
181. **Your Vital Papers Logbook.** *$4.95 / AARP member price $2.95.*
818. **Fitness for Life:** *Exercises for People Over 50. $12.95 / AARP member price $9.45.*
825. **A Woman's Guide to Good Health After 50.** *$12.95 / AARP member price $9.45.*
833. **On the Road in an RV.** *$8.95 / AARP member price $6.50.*

Join AARP today and enjoy valuable benefits

Join the American Association of Retired Persons, the national organization which helps people like you, age 50 and over, realize their full potential in so many ways! The rewards you'll reap with AARP will be many times greater than your low membership dues. And your membership also includes your spouse!

☐ START MY MEMBERSHIP IN AARP

- ☐ one year/$5
- ☐ three years/$12.50 (saves $2.50)
- ☐ ten years/$35 (saves $15)

- ☐ Check or money order enclosed, payable to AARP. DO NOT SEND CASH
- ☐ Please bill me

Name (please print)

Address _____ Apt.

City

State _____ Zip

Date of Birth _____ mo/ _____ day/ _____ year

☐ *Start my membership in NRTA (a division for those in or retired from education)*

Information You Can Count On!

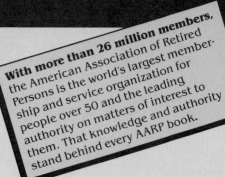

With more than 26 million members, the American Association of Retired Persons is the world's largest membership and service organization for people over 50 and the leading authority on matters of interest to them. That knowledge and authority stand behind every AARP book.

832. **The Sleep Book:** Understanding and Preventing Sleep Problems in People Over 50. *$10.95 / AARP member price $7.95.*

822. **Sunbelt Retirement:** The Complete State-by-State Guide. *$11.95 / AARP member price $8.50.*

824. **Walking for the Health of It.** The Easy and Effective Exercise for People Over 50. *$6.95 / AARP member price $4.95.*

826. **Think of Your Future.** Retirement Planning Workbook. *$24.95 / AARP member price $18.25.*

HOW TO ORDER

To order state book name and number, quantity and price (AARP members: be sure to include your membership no. for discount) and add $1.75 *per entire order* for shipping and handling. *All orders must be prepaid.* For your convenience we accept checks, money orders, VISA and MasterCard (credit card orders must include card no., exp. date and cardholder signature). *Please allow 4 weeks for delivery.*

Send your order today to:
AARP Books / Scott, Foresman and Co., 1865 Miner Street
Des Plaines, IL 60016

AARP Books are co-published by AARP and Scott, Foresman and Co., sold by Scott, Foresman and Co., and distributed to bookstores by Little, Brown and Company.

Join AARP today and enjoy valuable benefits

65% of dues is designated for Association publications. Dues outside continental U.S.: $7 one year, $18 three years. Please allow 3 to 6 weeks for receipt of membership kit.

NO POSTAGE
NECESSARY
IF MAILED
IN THE
UNITED STATES

BUSINESS REPLY MAIL
FIRST CLASS   PERMIT NO. 3132   LONG BEACH, CA

POSTAGE WILL BE PAID BY ADDRESSEE

American Association of Retired Persons
Membership Processing Center
P.O. Box 199
Long Beach, CA 90801-9989

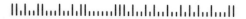